**Patterns**

**International Library of Sociology
and Social Reconstruction**

Founded by Karl Mannheim
Editor: W. J. H. Sprott

A catalogue of books available in the **International Library of Sociology and Social Reconstruction** and new books in preparation for the Library will be found at the end of this volume.

# Patterns of residential care
## Sociological studies in institutions for handicapped children

Roy D. King, Norma V. Raynes and
Jack Tizard

London   Routledge & Kegan Paul

First published in 1971
by Routledge and Kegan Paul Ltd,
Broadway House,
68–74 Carter Lane,
London EC4V 5EL
Printed in Great Britain
by Willmer Brothers Limited, Birkenhead
© Roy D. King, Norma V. Raynes
and Jack Tizard 1971
ISBN   0 7100 7038 1

# Contents

## Appendices

# Acknowledgments

The studies described in this monograph were carried out between 1963 and 1968. The investigations were made possible by a grant from the (American) Association for the Aid of Crippled Children. We are deeply grateful to the Association for its generous support. The grant was administered first by the Medical Research Council, and after 1964 by the University of London Institute of Education.

The fieldwork was carried out in more than one hundred separate living units in twenty-six different establishments for children. In some establishments we spent several months; in others only a week. In all of them we were received with kindness and tolerance in spite of the heavy burden which our research placed on our respondents. Our greatest debt, therefore, is to the staffs of the living units we studied, and to the administrators who were responsible for the establishments. A great many people, at all levels, put themselves out to make our studies rewarding, and without their ready co-operation we could not have completed our work. Though we cannot mention all of them by name, we are glad to acknowledge them here. In our comments we are sometimes critical of the manner in which establishments function. We should, however, be distressed if this were taken as a personal criticism of the staffs themselves. It would indeed indicate that the main point of our studies had not got across—namely that institutions differ in their patterns of care because they are differently organized, and because the structure of the organization acts as a constraint on what can be achieved. We did not ourselves inquire into the personal qualities of staff, nor were we attempting to judge them in any way as caretakers of children. But no one who has watched nursing staff and child care staff at work can fail to be impressed by what they see.

## ACKNOWLEDGMENTS

Many people have contributed to our work in different ways. We owe a special debt to Dr Stephen Richardson of the A.A.C.C. for his constant interest, criticism and advice. Dr George Brown and Dr Albert Kushlick have given us valuable suggestions, particularly on methods, many of which we have been happy to adopt. We would like to thank Mr William Yule, both for his work during the field studies when he was engaged on the project, and for his most helpful interest and advice subsequently. We are grateful to Mr Paul Williams, who allowed us to use some of the material he had collected for an undergraduate dissertation which related to one of the establishments we studied.

Among the many people who have given advice on specific problems, or who have contributed through discussion, are Miss Frances Cherry, Miss Gillian Cox, Professor Sir Aubrey Lewis, Dr I. Barry Pless, Professor Noel Timms and Dr J. K. Wing. For short periods during the studies, we were ably assisted in the coding and analysis of data by Mrs Brenda Denvir, Mrs Kate Fearnhead, Miss Maureen Hemmings, Mrs Janet King, Miss Vanessa Martin, Mrs Ahelia Noon, Mr Michael Stein, and Mr Robin Williams. Mrs Cassandra Williams, in addition to her secretarial duties, skilfully arranged for the smooth running of the field work in the survey. Other clerical assistance has been provided by Miss Ann Cossart and Miss Rae Eggby. Miss Olwen Davies, who acted as secretary to the Project, typed the first draft and prepared the index. Mrs Jo Bartlett coped with the many amendments to the text and typed the final draft.

Lastly, we are grateful to Dr Barbara Tizard, who read the final draft and offered many helpful suggestions and criticisms. Needless to say, we alone bear responsibility for the conduct of the studies and for the contents of this report.

R.D.K.
N.V.R.
J.T.

# part one

# Background to the studies

# 1 Introduction

This monograph describes a series of studies dealing with the up-bringing of children in residential institutions. Most of the work has been carried out in institutions for the mentally retarded, although units caring for normal, but deprived, children and for physically handicapped children have also been examined. The investigations have been concerned with the detailed nature of different institutional environments—that is, the routine patterns of daily life in hospital wards, hostels and cottages of children's homes—rather than with the effects of specific child-rearing practices upon the intellectual, emotional and social development of the children. The more precise delineation of 'the environment' is an essential step towards the evaluation of residential services and the interpretation of their effects upon those who use them, yet this is an area which has received little systematic attention from social scientists.

The unit for analysis throughout has been the individual ward or cottage in which the children live, and we have looked to the organizational structure of this unit and that of the wider institutional context in which it is found, for an explanation of the differences in daily patterns of care. We have chosen to examine such matters as institutional size and authority structure, staff–child ratios, the role activities of child care staff and the way they perform them, and staff training in so far as these relate to child management patterns, rather than, for example, the personality characteristics of staff who come and go, or staff attitudes towards children and their upbringing. The orientation is thus sociological rather than psychological.

Our focus on living units rather than children was dictated by our interest in the more generally persisting features of child care which characterize institutions of different types. We have tried to present the differences in patterns of care by the use of a simple scale, which measures some important elements of child management practice. Our choice of the organizational variables studied has reflected our preference for handling 'hard' data, relating to events which can be objectively and reliably measured and which have some stability over time. It follows that our approach has been avowedly quantitative, because we believe the use of quantitative techniques provides a more precise and systematic means of comparison than a straightforward description. We have not, however, divorced measurement from description, and we hope that the relationship between the descriptive and the quantitative aspects of our work will be self-evident. Together we believe them to provide a characterization of the quality of residential care for children.

## Origins of the study

In 1962 a grant was made to one of us (J.T.) to set up a research group to study 'patterns of child management and their effects upon the development of children from different social backgrounds, and of different ages, abilities, and handicaps, with special reference to upbringing in residential institutions'. It was intended from the outset that the research should be concerned with practical as well as theoretical issues. In applying for the grant, it was pointed out that no substantial reduction in the numbers of children who would spend all, or a substantial proportion, of their lives in residential institutions could be expected. Indeed, numbers were increasing—and they have continued to increase since that time, as Chapter 2 points out. Problems relating to the residential care of children were therefore of great practical importance, as well as being of lively theoretical interest to sociologists and psychologists.

At the time, it was evident that there existed great contrasts between different types of institutional care. The mentally retarded in particular were brought up in a manner which compared very unfavourably with that in which ordinary, non-handicapped children who were deprived of a normal home life were reared, either in residential nurseries for babies and infants, or in children's homes which serve mainly the needs of children of school age. Differences of this order were also to be found in other countries which provided for the mentally retarded: these differences persisted over time and could not be accounted for in terms of idiosyncratic features associated with individual establishments. Either they arose out of the nature of the retarded child's handicap—which necessitated a different type of regimen—or they resulted from differences in the social organization of the establishments.

There were several reasons for believing that organizational features are of primary importance in determining the type of care given to the mentally retarded. First, it was only during the preceding fifteen years that methods of bringing up *normal* children who were orphans or otherwise deprived of normal home care had changed dramatically. In England, at the end of the Second World War, conditions in workhouses and in children's institutions resembled, for the most part, the conditions which still obtained in mental deficiency hospitals. The Curtis Committee (1946) drew attention to the sad plight of children who were 'deprived of normal home life' and stirred the public conscience. A new Children Act of 1948 led to the establishment of a Children's Department as part of the Home Office, and all Local Authorities were required to set up Local Children's Departments, which were charged with the responsibility of providing adequate care for deprived ('dependent' in U.S. terminology) children. During the 1950s, a transformation of residential child care practices for ordinary children was effected (Heywood, 1959). Similar changes, brought about by the postwar concern for the welfare of children, occurred in other countries during the same period.

Second, during the 1950s a change in the organization of other types of residential institution was beginning to take place, with similar consequences. Many adult mental hospitals began to be organized in a new way, and more concern was shown in the welfare of mental patients with chronic handicaps. Active measures were introduced not merely to get patients out of hospitals as soon as possible, but to improve the quality of hospital life itself. The same process was beginning to be felt in other types of establishment, notably old people's homes.

Third, some experiments have shown that it *was* possible to bring up severely retarded children in a manner which resembled that followed in residential nurseries for normal pre-school children of about the same mental age. When this was done, the children benefited both socially and emotionally, as well as in terms of intellectual development (Tizard, 1964).

The evidence, then, showed that there was a wide variety of institutional practice. Institutions, and in particular large institutions, which had received most study, did not all conform to a common norm. More enlightened and less repressive measures than had been customary in the past were being introduced in a number of different kinds of establishments dealing with handicapped people—and when this happened, the results were indubitably good.

However, there had—and still have—been few comparative studies of institutions, and fewer still of children's institutions. Moreover, the studies which had been undertaken served more to demonstrate what achievements were feasible, than to show what organizational features were responsible for one type of care rather than another, and they failed to provide criteria for use in evaluating patterns of upbringing outside the family.

It was proposed to undertake a number of statistical, social and psychological studies into aspects of institutional care; and the American Association for the Aid of Crippled Children, to whom an application for funds was made, gave a generous grant over a five-year period in support of what we have called the Child Welfare Project.

## Progress of the research

The research was begun in 1963 when the two sociologists (R.D.K. and N.V.R.) were appointed to the project. Because we had to start the empirical research work from scratch, progress was at first slow. Three years were spent in defining aims and methods more precisely, and in developing quantitative scales by which to measure aspects of institutional functioning. During this period, we also undertook detailed field studies of two large children's homes for deprived normal children, a longstay children's hospital for chronic sick and physically handicapped children, and a mental deficiency hospital. At a slightly later date, a further investigation was carried out in two smaller institutions for mentally retarded children.

An account of these studies forms Part II of this monograph. The evidence gained supported our general view that it was the social organization of the establishment, rather than the handicaps of the children, which was primarily responsible for differences in child management practices between the two children's homes on the one hand, and the two hospitals on the other. However, the investigations raised further questions, and to examine these we subsequently undertook a larger study of sixteen institutions, all of them serving the needs of mentally retarded children. The purposes were: (1) to examine much more carefully child management practices in a large number of institutions, all of them dealing with the same type of child; (2) to explore relations among different aspects of institutional structure and functioning; (3) to relate child management practices to aspects of institutional organization. This work is described in detail in Part III. It represents the first stage in the task of systematic description of the working and effectiveness of residential institutions for children.

Part I sets out the background for the research in terms of the numbers of children in different forms of care, and reviews recent theory and research in residential institutions. In the last section, Part IV, we discuss the implications of the investigations and present some conclusions.

# 2    Children in residential care

## The size of the problem

Because responsibility for the care and upbringing of handicapped, deprived and delinquent children is divided among a number of different authorities, and because there is no uniform system of statistical returns, it is not easy to say how many children are in residential care at any one time, or how many spend different periods of time away from their families in substitute forms of care. The problem is not confined to Britain: to obtain national statistics from countries on the continent of Europe or North America, for example, is equally difficult.*

In England, the first and most thorough inquiry 'directed specifically to the care of children deprived of a normal home life, and covering all groups of such children' was that undertaken by the Curtis Committee (1946). At that time there were nearly 125,000 children who were 'deprived' of normal home life, being brought up in some form of residential care. Table 2.1 shows how these children were distributed among the different forms of available substitute care, and who was responsible for their upbringing.

Over the next two decades the administrative pattern of services for children changed greatly, a new emphasis being placed on preventive measures, but the numbers of children receiving some form of residential care none the less increased from about 125,000 in 1946 to over 146,000 in 1963. An indication of the size of the problem may be gained by comparing the numbers in care with those in school sixth forms or at universities. In January 1963 the total number of pupils in all sixth forms in England and Wales was 136,253 (*Statistics of Education,* 1966), and in 1963-4 there

* Personal communication, Dr G. Dybwad.

8

were only 116,000 full-time students in universities in England and Wales (Layard *et al.*, 1969).*

TABLE 2.1   *Children deprived of a normal home life, 1946*[a]

| Category | Disposal | Number | Total |
|---|---|---|---|
| 1 Deprived children | In care of Local Authorities<br>In care of voluntary orgs. | 40,900[b]<br>26,700[c] | 67,600 |
| 2 Protected children | In foster homes, for reward<br>In foster homes, for adoption | 10,700<br>2,400 | 13,100 |
| 3 Delinquent children | In approved schools<br>In remand homes<br>In probation homes and hostels | 11,200<br>1,500<br>700 | 13,400 |
| 4 Handicapped children (in special schools) | In Local Authority special schools<br>In special schools run by voluntary orgs. | 6,300<br>8,200 | 14,500 |
| 5 Handicapped children (in other institutions) | In hospitals or boarded out<br>In care of voluntary orgs. | 7,200<br>300[d] | 7,500 |
| 6 Homeless evacuees and war orphans | In Local Authority homes<br>In voluntary orgs.<br>In foster homes | 1,900<br>300<br>6,600 | 8,800 |
| All categories | | 124,900 | 124,900 |

[a]Adapted from Table IV, p. 27, *The Curtis Report* (Cmnd 6922).
[b]This figure includes 4,600 children in voluntary homes but chargeable to the Poor Law, and 8,000 children removed from home by the courts.
[c]Includes 2,000 children removed from home by the courts.
[d]This does not include uncertified children, for whom no figures are available.

As in 1946, so in 1963 the largest group of children in residential care were 'deprived' children, but the pattern of Poor Law Administration had, by that time, been replaced. The 1948 Children Act created a Local Authority Children's Service for the specific purpose of caring for children who, either permanently or temporarily, were deprived of a normal home life. The new service unified and greatly improved the patchwork of services still existing at the end of the Second World War. In March 1963 there were 64,807 children in the care of Local Authorities, some 3,714 of them being

* It should be added that during the last seven years the number of full-time university students and the number of sixth-form pupils have both increased greatly, while no corresponding increase in the numbers of children in care has occurred, so that this comparison no longer holds.

B

boarded by Local Authorities in homes run by voluntary organizations. These voluntary bodies themselves maintained a further 13,218 children. An additional 8,038 children were maintained for reward in private foster homes and institutions, and a further 6,988 children were awaiting adoption by people other than their parents.

Next in size came the group of handicapped children educated in special residential schools. Of course, not all special schools are boarding establishments, and many boarding schools also take day pupils. In January 1963 there were 22,846 pupils in special boarding schools, of whom 20,579 were boarders and 2,267 attending on a day basis. There were, in addition, a number of other independent boarding schools, many of them specializing in the care and education of maladjusted children. In 1963 these schools accommodated 3,105 children, bringing the total number of handicapped pupils boarding in special schools to 23,684.

Delinquent children come into something of a special category in that accommodation is required for them as a result of the jurisdiction of the courts. However, the younger delinquent groups came within the terms of reference of the Curtis Committee in 1946 and these groups may be usefully considered here. It is in any case likely that many delinquent children share the same characteristics as deprived children who come into care of the Local Authorities in the ordinary way. Indeed, the legal distinction between the deprived and the delinquent has been progressively diminished over the years, so that under the provisions of the Children and Young Persons Act, 1969, both groups will, in future, normally be dealt with through care proceedings. Most delinquent children in residential accommodation are in 'approved schools'—that is, schools which are specially approved by the Secretary of State as being suitable boarding establishments for the delinquent. In 1963 there were 121 such schools, of which 93 were managed by voluntary organizations. In all, they cared for 8,535 children, of whom 7,382 were boys. Some 580 children were in approved probation homes and hostels, and a further 1,232 boys and girls were in remand homes, usually awaiting consideration by the juvenile courts or allocation to other institutions.

Most of these delinquents were children or young persons under the age of sixteen. A further 5,930 young persons who had been convicted by the courts and who were in detention centres or Borstals in 1963 have been excluded from Table 2.2: for the most part they were over the age of sixteen and their counterparts in 1946 had not been considered by the Curtis Committee.

The last major category of children in residential care comprised those who are mentally or physically handicapped to such a degree that they cannot be accommodated in residential special schools. It is difficult to give the total numbers in this group because of the inadequacy of officially published statistics, but it is probable that in 1963 there were between 15,000 and 19,000 such children. There were 4,091 physically handicapped or sick children in hospital schools; 1,595 children and young persons under the age of twenty in hospitals for the mentally ill; 13,127 in hospitals and homes for the subnormal; and 286 in Local Authority hostels for the subnormal.

A more detailed account of the numbers of children in various forms of care, and of the sources from which the statistics have been taken, has been given by King (1970). Table 2.2 summarizes the statistics.

To compare the statistics for 1963 with those for 1946 is scarcely

TABLE 2.2   *Children deprived of a normal home life, 1963*[a]

| Category | Disposal | Number | Total |
|----------|----------|--------|-------|
| 1 Deprived children | In care of Local Authorities | 64,807 | 78,025 |
| | In care of voluntary org'ns | 13,218[b] | |
| 2 Protected children | In foster homes, for reward | 8,038 | 15,026 |
| | In foster homes, for adoption | 6,988 | |
| 3 Delinquent children | In approved schools | 8,535 | 10,347 |
| | In remand homes | 1,232 | |
| | In probation homes and hostels | 580 | |
| 4 Handicapped children (in special schools) | In Local Authority maintained special schools | 12,980 | 23,684 |
| | In non-maintained special schools | 7,599 | |
| | In other independent schools | 3,105[c] | |
| 5 Handicapped children (in other institutions) | In hospital schools (physically ill) | 4,091 | 19,099 |
| | In hospitals (mentally ill) | 1,595 | |
| | In hospitals and homes (subnormal) | 13,127 | |
| | In Local Authority hostels (subnormal) | 286 | |
| All categories | | 146,181 | 146,181 |

[a]Adapted from Table 1.2, King (1970).
[b]This figure excludes 3,714 in care of Local Authorities and boarded in voluntary organizations. It also excludes children in their own homes receiving financial aid from voluntary sources.
[c]These children are not in 'special schools' in the technical sense, but are similar to those who do attend special schools.

11

a profitable undertaking. It is likely that the Curtis Committee omitted certain groups of children who have been included in the 1963 figures. Even so, the increases in absolute numbers could be accounted for by a variety of factors: changes in the law; changes in the administration of services, including a more adequate system of ascertaining needs and a better system of record keeping; and, not the least, changes in the age structure of the total population. The change in age structure is particularly important. Donnison and Ungerson (1968), for example, using data from census returns, have shown that although absolute numbers of persons (of all ages) in residential care increased greatly between 1911 and 1961, when the size and demographic structure of the population are taken into account by the calculation of age-specific in-care rates, the proportions of persons in each age group cared for in residential institutions can be seen to have declined.

For children, the rise in numbers between 1946 and 1966 was by no means a regular one: following the passing of the Children Act in 1948, the number of children in the care of Local Authorities rose to a peak of 65,000 in 1953 and thereafter declined to 61,000 in 1959. At that point, numbers increased again to nearly 65,000 in 1963 and reached a new peak of 69,000 in 1966. Expressed as rates per thousand of the estimated total population under the age of eighteen years, however, the 1953 peak represents a higher proportion of children in care than does the peak in 1966. In-care rates were respectively 5·6 in 1953, 5·1 in 1959, 5·1 in 1963 and 5·3 in 1966. Moreover, the absolute increase in Local Authority provision was matched by a decrease in the numbers of children in the care of voluntary organizations. These fell from 20,153 in 1954 to 17,068 in 1959, 13,218 in 1963 and to 10,839 in 1966. Combining the two groups, the downward trend is marked and regular: from 7·6 per thousand in 1953-4 to 6·5 in 1959, 6·4 in 1963 and 6·1 in 1966.* It should be added that about half the children admitted to care today are shortstay cases, although these make up only about 7 per cent of those in care at any one time.

### The quality of residential care

With changes in the organization of residential care for children have come changes in its nature. Children who require substitute care come from different social backgrounds and present different ranges of handicaps and abilities, and the authorities responsible for providing care have differing traditions and differing means at

* See *Children in the Care of Local Authorities in England and Wales*, 1953–4, 1959, 1963, 1966; also Packman (1968).

their disposal. In consequence it is perhaps inevitable that the type and quality of provision should still vary considerably. It is still unfortunately true that improvements in one field have not always been carried over into others; and though all forms of residential care have improved in quality during the last fifteen to twenty years, some types of care have been radically restructured, whereas others have merely been 'upgraded'. A brief account of changes affecting the care of deprived children on the one hand, and mentally handicapped children on the other, illustrates the manner in which changes have taken place in contrasting types of care.

*Deprived children*

At the time of the Curtis Report (1946), most deprived children were still accommodated under the provisions of the Poor Law Act, 1930, as persons in need of relief. The administration of these services was mainly under the general direction of the Ministry of Health and the Local Authorities who normally acted through Public Assistance Committees. Accommodation was mainly of two types: 'barrack homes', which were large, self-contained, residential establishments usually consisting of a single building, and technically known as 'separate schools'; and 'grouped cottage homes', which consisted of several houses occupying the same site and together making a larger children's community. A few children were accommodated in what were called 'scattered homes', or single houses on ordinary residential estates. In addition, there were nearly as many children not under the Poor Law, in homes of the same three types, which were administered by voluntary organizations. Comparatively few children were 'boarded out' in foster homes, and a few were actually living in workhouses.

The Curtis Committee (1946) was extremely critical of the services which it examined. It was 'far from satisfied with the immediate provision made for children coming as destitute or in need of care or protection into the care of Local Authorities'. Too often, reception arrangements consisted of placing the child into a 'workhouse ward, where there is nothing but the barest provision for his physical needs, and where the staff have neither the capacity nor the time to relieve his fears, make him feel at ease, or give him occupation or interest' (para. 415). The Committee was shocked, not so much by the standards of physical care, as by the 'dirt and dreariness, drabness and over-regimentation' of many establishments:

We did find many establishments under both local authority and voluntary management in which children were being brought

13

up by unimaginative methods, without opportunity for developing their full capabilities and with very little brightness or interest in their surroundings. We found, in fact, many places where the standard of child care was no better, except in respect of disciplinary methods, than that of, say, 30 years ago; and we found a widespread and deplorable shortage of the right kind of staff, personally qualified and trained to provide the children with a substitute for a home background. The result in many homes was a lack of personal interest in, and affection for, the children, which we found shocking. The child in these homes was not recognized as an individual, with his own rights and possessions, his own life to live and his own contribution to offer. He was merely one of a large crowd, eating, playing and sleeping with the rest, without any place or possession of his own, or any quiet room to which he could retreat. Still more important, he was without the feeling that there was anyone to whom he could turn who was vitally interested in his welfare or who cared for him as a person [para. 418].

In part, the buildings and equipment of many homes could be blamed for these conditions. The Report deplored the 'large, gaunt-looking buildings with dark stairways and corridors, high windows and unadapted baths and lavatories' which were found not only among workhouses run by local authorities, but also among 'barrack' homes run by Public Assistance Committees and by some voluntary organizations. But more important than mere buildings were shortages of staff and their lack of training, and the poor co-operation between the central authorities and the local management.

In their examination of the practice of boarding out children in foster homes, the Committee found that the children were, for the most part, free from the sense of deprivation that was so prevalent among the children in homes. Foster homes as a whole 'made a remarkably favourable impression' on the Committee, although closer supervision by trained staff was deemed to be essential. The Report added that 'there is probably a greater risk of acute unhappiness in a foster home, but that a happy foster home is happier than life as generally lived in a large community' (paras. 420-2).

As already mentioned the Curtis Report recommended that ultimate responsibility for deprived children should be with one central Government Department, the actual provision of services remaining a matter for Local Authorities and voluntary organizations, who would, in future, have to be registered with the central Department. Standards of care and supervision would be maintained and improved by the powers of inspection and discretion to be vested in the new Department. It seemed to the Committee that boarding out provided the best method, after adoption, of giving a deprived child a satisfactory substitute home, and it was therefore recommended that, given suitable safeguards, the practice should be greatly extended. The Report recognized, however, that it would be impossible to foster all children, and that the need for institutional care must be faced, with the aim of 'making it as good a substitute for the private home as it can possibly be' (para. 476).

To minimize the disadvantages of institutional life, it was recommended first that children should be placed in institutions which were quite separate from adult institutions; second, that babies and young infants should be cared for in specialized residential nurseries; third, that the pattern of care in all cases should be constructed so as to resemble as closely as possible that found in normal families (paras. 478-89).

The family pattern of care was to be achieved by placing a child at the earliest possible age in a small group of children of various ages and both sexes, under the care of a trained and sympathetic housemother, or housemother and housefather. The small group home should contain not more than twelve children, although eight was the preferred size, and, wherever possible, brothers and sisters should be kept in the same family unit. 'Scattered homes' in residential areas, where the children could attend normal schools, seemed the best alternative after fostering, although the Committee agreed that much had been and could be done within the group cottage homes. Where large barrack homes were still unavoidably in use, every effort should be made to subdivide them, so that a family group system could be introduced.

The Curtis Report had an immediate and profound effect on public policy. Legislation followed in 1948, setting up the Children's Department of the Home Office. The proportion of children in the care of Local Authorities who were boarded out rose from 35 per cent in 1949 to 42 per cent in 1953, 47 per cent in 1959 and 52 per cent in 1963. In 1966, the proportion fell to 50·5 per cent, because of the rapid increase in the numbers coming into care and the difficulties of obtaining foster placements; even so, the numbers boarded out in that year were greater than ever before in absolute terms.

Along with this increase in boarding out, there was steady progress in closing down larger establishments, particularly the older and more gloomy ones. These have been replaced by smaller, scattered homes, run on a family group basis. By 1966, three-fifths of all the homes, nurseries and hostels run by Local Authorities were 'small' homes, and only one-fifth had been in use 'for a similar purpose' before 1948. Between 1953 and 1966, the number of children accommodated in small homes had doubled from 3,676 to 7,126, while the number in other children's homes, excluding reception homes and nurseries, had almost halved from 14,699 to 7,822. A similar pattern of development has taken place in the voluntary organizations caring for deprived children.

Large homes still exist in both Local Authority and voluntary provision, but strenuous efforts have been made to reform them in accordance with the Curtis Committee recommendations. Thus, buildings have been partitioned, and houseparents have been given greater independence, to allow them to form family groups within existing structures. Even in the largest units, much has been done to increase the children's sense of belonging and personal identity, through the provision of personal possessions and individualized clothing and the fostering of close links with the surrounding community.*

## Mentally handicapped children in hospital

Changes during the last twenty-five years in the patterns of care for the mentally handicapped have been less radical. Since the Second World War there have been major administrative changes, which have included the coming into being of the National Health Service in 1948, and the implementation of a new and comprehensive Mental Health Act in 1960. These have markedly affected the administrative organization of services; but nothing comparable to the Curtis Committee review of services for deprived children has been undertaken—at least until 1969 when the Department of Health and Social Security set up a Working Party on Services for the subnormal. Earlier, there had been a number of specialized enquiries, or reports, of which the Scott Committee Report on the training of teachers of the mentally handicapped and a Departmental circular on improving the effectiveness of the hospital service for the subnormal (H.M.[65] 104) were the most important. In 1962, a policy statement 'A Hospital Plan for England and Wales' (Cmnd 1064) was published, giving guidance to authorities on the type of accommodation recommended for the mentally handicapped.

Residential care for those mentally subnormal persons who require it is, in Britain as in most other countries, usually provided in mental subnormality hospitals, and something should be said of the characteristics of this hospital population. Since the Mental Health Act of 1960, which made voluntary admission to and discharge from hospital the rule rather than the exception, the num-

* See *Reports on the Work of the Children's Department*, 1955–66.

bers of patients admitted and discharged have increased markedly. Whereas in 1954 there were fewer than 3,000 patients a year admitted to mental subnormality hospitals in 1968 the number had increased to nearly 11,000. In 1968 also, nearly 10,000 patients were discharged, two-thirds of them within three months of admission ('shortstay cases') and more than three-quarters in less than one year. The majority of those discharged (other than those who came into hospital specifically in order to relieve some temporary family crisis or to give parents a rest, or a holiday) are mildly subnormal young persons or adults; few severely subnormal persons, whether children or adults, leave hospital once they have been admitted for other than short-term care, and at any one time the great majority of patients would have been in hospital for years rather than months, and will remain there until they die.

The *sex and age* distribution of patients in mental subnormality hospitals in 1964 can be judged from figures collected by Morris (1969). Her data are reproduced in Table 2.3.

TABLE 2.3   *Percentage sex and age distribution of patients in hospital sample, Morris, (1969)*[a]

| Age group (years) | Male | Female | Total | Estimated total population, England and Wales 1964* |
|---|---|---|---|---|
| 0–4 | 1·1 | 1·1 | 1·1 | 8·4 |
| 5–9 | 4·5 | 3·8 | 4·2 | 7·2 |
| 10–15 | 7·3 | 6·1 | 6·8 | 8·5 |
| 16–19 | 8·5 | 6·8 | 7·7 | 6·3 |
| 20–29 | 19·5 | 15·6 | 17·7 | 12·9 |
| 30–39 | 16·7 | 13·9 | 15·5 | 12·7 |
| 40–49 | 16·3 | 17·4 | 16·8 | 13·0 |
| 50–59 | 15·4 | 17·9 | 16·5 | 13·1 |
| 60 and over | 10·7 | 17·4 | 13·8 | 17·6 |
| Total | 100·0 | 100·0 | 100·0 | 100·0 |
| No information | 16 | 14 | 30 | — |
| No. of persons | 1,664 | 1,374 | 3,038 | 47,511,000 |

* Source: Registrar-General's Statistical Review of England and Wales for the year 1964.
[a]Taken from Table 4.1, p. 61, Morris (1969).

As the table indicates, there are somewhat more males than females in hospital. A higher proportion of females are in the older age groups, but males still outnumber females in every age group except those aged sixty and over. Only about 12 per cent of the patients are children under the age of sixteen, and nearly all of these are severely subnormal.

The best information regarding the distribution of *handicaps* in the patient population comes from a survey carried out by Kushlick and Cox in 1963 in the Wessex region of southern England, an area with a total population of 1·8 million persons, and with 5,000 patients in residential institutions. The figures for this region accord pretty well with those found elsewhere in the country, as far as is known.

Kushlick and Cox (1968, 1970) divided patients by grade of defect into two groups, *severely subnormal patients,* being those with IQ less than 50, and *mildly subnormal patients,* namely those with IQ of 50 and above. The handicaps of the patients were defined in functional terms, four groups being distinguished. These were non-ambulance (NA); severe behaviour disorders (BD); severe incontinence (Inc.); and mild handicaps—that is, those with minor handicaps in one or more of the above, but without any severe handicaps. The figures given in Table 2·4 are taken from Kushlick and Cox (personal communication).

As the table shows, about 30 per cent of the children were non-ambulant, and a further 25 per cent had severe behaviour disorders, with or without severe incontinence; about 45 per cent were ambulant children who did not present severe behaviour disorders, though about a third of these were severely incontinent, and fewer than half presented neither major nor minor problems.

The figures for adults were very different. Only about 6 per cent of the adults were non-ambulant, the majority of these being severely subnormal patients. About the same proportion suffered from severe incontinence, but were ambulant. The proportion of patients who had severe behaviour disorders was about 14 per cent, the majority of them severely rather than mildly subnormal; most of them were continent. Three-quarters of the adult patients were continent, ambulant and without major behaviour disorders, and though somewhat over half these patients were severely retarded, as a group they presented rather minor problems of nursing or management. It is generally agreed, indeed, that large numbers of these patients could be discharged to other forms of residential care —if such places could be found for them in the community.

At the end of 1968 there were still about 65,000 mentally handicapped persons in hospitals, of whom 4,000 were in psychiatric hospitals, 800 in general hospitals, 2,600 in hospitals for the elderly, 900 in special hospitals for violent and dangerous defectives (Rampton and Moss Side Hospitals), and 58,000 in hospitals for the mentally subnormal. Many of these hospitals, transferred from Local Authorities into the National Health Service Hospital Service in 1948, were originally built for other purposes, or as public assistance institutions. About a fifth were built a century or more ago, and two-fifths before the turn of this century (Department of Health and Social Security—unpublished).

About three-quarters of the mentally handicapped are in forty-five hospitals with 500 or more beds, and about a third of them are in ten hospitals with 1,500 or more beds. Most of these hospitals, and in particular the larger and older ones, were built in rural areas—which makes both visiting, and the recruitment of staff, difficult. Many of the hospitals are greatly overcrowded, and there are long waiting lists for admission. In 1969, only 9 per cent of

TABLE 2.4   *Numbers of patients in mental deficiency hospitals with various types of handicap[a]*
*(Rates per 1,000 patients)*

| Type of patient | Type of handicap | | | | | | |
|---|---|---|---|---|---|---|---|
| | NA | Inc.+BD | BD | Inc. | Mild | None | Total |
| *Children* | | | | | | | |
| S.S.N. | 37 | 20 | 11 | 19 | 12 | 21 | 120 |
| M.S.N. | 2 | 1 | 2 | 0 | 2 | 4 | 12 |
| All | 39 | 21 | 13 | 20 | 14 | 25 | 133 |
| *Adults* | | | | | | | |
| S.S.N. | 42 | 26 | 64 | 39 | 81 | 273 | 525 |
| M.S.N. | 11 | 2 | 27 | 5 | 32 | 266 | 343 |
| All | 53 | 28 | 91 | 44 | 113 | 539 | 868 |
| Total | 92 | 49 | 104 | 64 | 127 | 564 | 1000 |

NA = Non-ambulant
Inc. = Severely incontinent
BD = Having a severe behaviour disorder
Mild = Having a mild handicap of mobility and/or behaviour and/or incontinence but no severe handicap.
None = None of the above
S.S.N. = Severely subnormal (IQ < 50)
M.S.N. = Mildly subnormal (IQ 50+)
[a]Taken from unpublished data supplied by Kushlick and Cox (personal communication). The rates are calculated from population data on 2,904 patients in Wessex mental subnormality hospitals on whom there was full information. Twenty-seven patients whose grade of mental handicap was not known, and forty-six on whom there was insufficient information regarding handicaps, have been omitted from the analysis.

beds were in dormitories with 70 or more square feet per bed, and only 9 per cent of patients were in wards which had reached the recommended desirable minimum standard of 48 or more square feet of day space per patient. There were less than 50 square feet per bed available in the dormitories in which nearly 60 per cent of the patients slept, and more than 80 per cent of patients were housed in wards with less than 40 square feet per patient available in the day rooms (Department of Health and Social Security—unpublished). A detailed description of mental deficiency institutions has recently been published by Morris (1969).

Over a fourteen-year period (between 1954 and 1968) there was, however, a steady improvement in hospital conditions. The average number of daily occupied beds in hospitals for the subnormal in 1954 was 51,356; there were 8,041 nurses ('whole-time equivalents') available to look after them. By 1968, the number of patients had risen to 58,217, and the number of nurses to 14,114. Thus, between 1954 and 1968, the population of patients rose by 4,861, while the number of nurses increased by 6,073: the patient to staff ratio fell from 6:6 in 1954 to 4:1 in 1968 (Department of Health and Social Security—unpublished).

*Residential care of the mentally handicapped 'in the community'*

The most important developments in residential care for the mentally handicapped during the last ten years have come from the extension of Local Authority and other 'community' services. Local Authorities have, for many years, had the responsibility of providing day services for mentally handicapped persons living in their own homes: welfare and medical services for families, education in day training centres for retardates of school age, sheltered workshops for retarded young people and adults, supervision and social work with the mentally handicapped of all ages and their families. These services have never been fully adequate, though in recent years provision has greatly increased, particularly for children.

The Royal Commission on the Law Relating to Mental Illness and Mental Deficiency, which reported in 1957, recommended a reorientation of services for the mentally handicapped away from institutional care in its existing form, and towards community care. Hospitals should provide in-patient and out-patient services for those needing specialist medical treatment or training, or continual nursing attention; Local Authorities should be responsible for those no longer requiring hospital treatment or training or who, after a period in hospital, were ready to return to the community. It was recognized that this would require great expansion of

Local Authority services to include residential accommodation in small homes or hostels for adults and children, more training facilities for children and school leavers, more occupational training centres or sheltered workshops for adults, and more social support for the handicapped of all ages and their families (Department of Health and Social Security—unpublished). In 1959, Local Health Authorities were given the duty to provide residential care (as well as other forms of community care) for the mentally handicapped. Since then they have been gradually developing this part of their services. By the end of 1968 they had provided, mostly by new building, sixty-four homes for children, containing 1,200 places. Many of these are used as boarding homes, five days a week, for children attending training centres who live too far away to travel daily. Local Authorities also maintain about 500 children in homes run by voluntary organizations or private individuals, and about sixty in private households. Similar arrangements are made for adults, of whom about 3,500 are cared for in this way. There are also about 1,700 mentally handicapped adults under the age of sixty-five, living in homes for the elderly, or other accommodation provided by Local Authorities through their welfare services. There are plans to build hostels providing 600 new places for children, and 2,000 new places for adults by March 1972. However, the majority of Local Authorities still make no provision of this sort.

Although the Local Authorities have, up to 1969, provided nearly 3,000 places in new residential homes and hostels for the mentally handicapped, and have found suitable homes elsewhere for another 2,000, only a small and uneven start has been made towards the objective of providing suitable residential care for all who need it but who do not need specialist medical and nursing care in hospital. Hospitals are still being called on to fulfil a social welfare as well as a medical function, and are having the greatest difficulty in doing either successfully (Department of Health and Social Security—unpublished).

## Discussion

The evolution of services for the mentally handicapped is following a pattern which is strikingly similar to that followed by the services for 'deprived' children after the Curtis Report of 1946. First, there is a new emphasis on 'preventive' services, the object of which is to provide for families services which will enable them to keep handicapped persons at home whenever possible. The need for this becomes greater as the quality of *residential* services improves—if good residential services are provided, but there is

21

little in the way of day services, families who keep a handicapped child at home actually deny him the services which he would receive if he were to be admitted to hospital. In these circumstances, even families who would otherwise willingly cope with the problems of caring for a retardate are forced to seek institutional care, since it is the only way in which the handicapped person can obtain services which would be his by right if he were an ordinary child (Tizard, 1964).

Second, much more is being done to encourage families to seek short-term care in times of crisis. The traditional attitude towards institutional care (for the deprived as well as the handicapped child) was to provide only longstay accommodation. Virtually all mentally subnormal 'patients' were legally detained in institutions until the passing of the Mental Health Act in 1959. Admission had to be preceded by 'certification' or committal proceedings, and parents lost their legal rights over their children. Today, admission is largely informal and there are many more admissions to care for short periods. It is recognized that it is a mistaken policy to have two independent services, one dealing with residential provision and the other with day services. Integration is required.

Third, there are growing moves to separate entirely the residential services for children from those for adults. The new hostel-type provision is specifically designed either for children or for adults; and in existing mental subnormality hospitals, which mostly take patients of all ages, the children's wards are separate from adult wards.

Fourth, the size of living units in institutions is being reduced. In 1965 the Department of Health advised that wards should not normally accommodate more than thirty adult patients or twenty children, and recommended that they should, wherever possible, be divided into smaller units. In 1962 it was suggested that patients who were not severely handicapped should be cared for in small units of not more than 200 beds, in areas with access to training facilities. The following year it was recommended that hospitals which catered for both the mildly and the severely subnormal should not have more than 500 beds. We are still a long way from reaching this standard; but the intention is there.

Fifth, there is less segregation of the sexes today. Segregation by sex is indeed still general in mental subnormality hospitals: 'There is little doubt that apart from young children's wards, when the sexes are often mixed, the only factor which receives *effective* consideration is that of sex' (Morris, 1969, p. 81). However, nearly all the new hostels, both for children and for adults, take retardates of both sexes — and more and more wards in general mental hospitals are being adapted so that they can take both men and women patients,

22

who share diningroom and day facilities, but who have separate sleeping accommodation.

Sixth, within the large barrack-type hospitals which are a legacy of the past, more money is being spent on 'upgrading'. The large, gaunt-looking buildings with dark stairways and corridors, high windows and unadapted baths and lavatories, of which the Curtis Committee complained, still exist in many mental subnormality hospitals. But some efforts have already been made to improve them, and more will be made in the future.

The mental subnormality services today are changing—and it is hoped that they will change more rapidly in the near future. The developments are similar to those which have occurred in other social services: the children's services, the mental hospital service, services for the old, and other welfare services for the handicapped.

It is difficult to say how far the developments in other services have influenced the changes in policy in the mental subnormality services, since there has been remarkably little collaboration between people responsible for various specialized services. What seems to have happened, not only this country but in Europe, North America and other parts of the word, is somewhat akin to what happened during the nineteenth century. 'After millennia of inactivity, the second half of the 1840s and the following decades witnessed the opening of one institution after another. As Seguin put it once: "At certain times and eras, the whole race of man, as regards the discovery of truth, seems to arrive at once at a certain point" ' (Kanner, 1964, p. 49).

It must not be forgotten, however, that the mental subnormality services do present problems which are not experienced by those who are responsible for services for socially deprived children. Many mentally handicapped persons have both physical and mental disabilities. They require more supervision, and for longer periods, than do normal children. The chronicity of mental handicap leads to different attitudes and expectations on the part of those who care for them. The attitudes of the public are also very different, as Wolfensberger (1969) has documented in an excellent and thorough review of mental deficiency hospital policy in the United States during the last century. (See also Davies, 1939; Kanner, 1964.) Official policy today acknowledges that the mentally retarded are handicapped persons who have a *right* to services, which society has a *duty* to provide. This attitude is quite new—indeed, in this country, the Mental Health Act of 1959 was the first to give legal expression to it, and full administrative expression can only come during the 1970s. The punitive or neglectful attitudes of the past have left a legacy of the old buildings, poor facilities, understaffing, overcrowding, inadequate provision of all sorts, and a lack of elementary amenities in the niggardly provision which has been made, so that it will be difficult to change or make good. Yet similar difficulties were rapidly overcome in large part by Local Authority Children's Departments twenty years ago, and comparable changes could rapidly occur in the mental health services also.

# 3 Child development and methods of upbringing

In the previous chapter, an account was given of some developments in the provision of residential services for handicapped and deprived children. Before describing our own empirical studies of the way in which these services function, something should be said about the current research on the upbringing of children in residential care, and about the substantial body of research which has been carried out on the residential institution as a form of complex organization. This chapter comments on research concerned with child development; the next on work in residential institutions.

Research on the upbringing of children in substitute types of care forms part of a larger field of study, namely that dealing with the effects of 'the environment' upon development. In one way or another, all developmental psychologists are concerned with this problem. The literature is immense, and the subject is already much over-reviewed. Our own treatment, therefore, will be brief and highly selective.

At least three sets of problems have been extensively studied. The first concerns the relative effects of heredity and environment upon cognitive development, and especially intelligence; the second is concerned with the effects of educational 'enrichment' upon school performance; and the third with the effects of what has come to be called 'maternal deprivation' upon personality and behaviour. In all three areas, some attention has been paid by investigators to the effects of institutional upbringing upon development.

## Genetic and environmental influences on intelligence

The heredity versus environment battle over the IQ, which had reached a stalemate following two sets of prolonged artillery ex-

C

changes in the 1920s and 1940s (reported in the *27th* and *39th Year Books of the National Society for the Study of Education*), has recently flared up again following an explosion set off by Jensen (1969) in a review of determinants of IQ. A debate on this topic now fills successive issues of the *Harvard Educational Review*. Sober accounts of the main points of controversy had already been presented and discussed well before the present bout of hostilities began (see, for example, Anastasi and Foley (1949); Clarke, 1965; Hunt, 1961; Huntley, 1966; Vernon, 1955; Woodworth, 1941). The exercises now being carried out for the most part merely repeat, though in a more sophisticated style, highly practised and familiar manoeuvres.

To a *social* scientist, what is so striking about much of this debate on the determinants of intelligence is not the passion with which it is conducted—which is explicable in political rather than scientific terms, as Pastore (1949) neatly pointed out some time ago. Nor is it the futility which arises because of the unsatisfactory and over-simplified models which have been used to elucidate the problems—as Haldane pointed out in the 1930s and 1940s, and as statistical analyses have later demonstrated (see, for example, Light and Smith (1969); and papers by Falconer and by Huntley in Meade and Parkes (1966)). Rather it is the bland and un-analytical way in which hereditarians and environmentalists alike use the word 'environment' as though it were a trait, like height, which varied along a single continuum, from great to small; from good to bad; from 'upper middle class' to 'lower working class'. Neither the justly renowned investigations into the beneficial effects of environmental changes upon IQ, carried out at the University of Iowa by Skeels and his collaborators during the 1930s (reviewed in Skeels, 1966), nor the meticulous and influential study of early education of the mentally retarded conducted by Kirk (1958) twenty years later, devote more than a paragraph or two to the conditions under which the children they studied were living, or the type of educational programme which they offered children in the 'experimental' situations. The attention of these investigators was focused on the children rather than on the social and educational environment; and while very detailed analyses were given of test findings obtained from the children, virtually no analysis was reported of experiential factors (including the educational programmes) which might have been responsible for gains or losses in 'intelligence'.

It was, of course, not unreasonable for Skeels and Kirk to have adopted this strategy. Skeels' work was, at the time, repudiated by psychologists (McNemar, 1940), and, as Guskin and Spicker (1968) point out, 'so entrenched was the belief that IQ scores were unmodifiable, that no serious attempt to demonstrate otherwise was made until Kirk conducted his study in the middle of the 1950s [p. 220]'. Given limited resources, therefore, the primary objective was naturally to demonstrate that in vastly different circumstances, children did develop differently. What may surprise future generations is that, in the middle of the twentieth century, this exercise should still have had to be carried out.

## The impact of 'compensatory' education

Research on 'compensatory' education, associated in the United States since 1965 with Project Headstart, has concentrated on curriculum development, and has also concerned itself very largely with the measurement of IQ and language change, and with the later educational progress and social adjustment of children in experimental and control groups. It is too hard to say, as Guskin and Spicker do in concluding an excellent review of work up to the end of 1967, that 'the current style of research has contributed pitifully little that is of value for the educational practitioner'. Nonetheless, these authors are right to point to its limitations. The upshot of compensatory programmes of education is a mean rise in IQ of about 5 to 15 points—and the rise is, in general, not sustained once the children move into the primary schools. Moreover, institutional children, who would seem to be those who would benefit most from compensatory education, have, if anything, benefited even less than children living in their own homes; and more handicapped children have made less progress than have brighter ones. There are many reasons for believing that this unsatisfactory state of affairs can be improved upon, not the least of them being the evidence obtained in the Skeels and Kirk studies. But progress will not come quickly; and it is apparent that further analysis of the *problem* is required.

There are several weaknesses in studies of compensatory education for the retarded. One is that bio-medical concomitants of retardation have received rather little attention from psychologists and educationalists. Kirk, for example, cites the greater intellectual and educational progress made by 'non-organic' children (that is, children who were retarded in intelligence but in whom no neurological handicaps could be diagnosed), than by a small group of 'organic' cases included in his pre-school study.

His numbers were very small, however, and the data he presents were not, in themselves, convincing. Moreover, whether or not Kirk's results were statistically significant is not the point; the statement that a child is 'organic' or 'brain injured' is not a useful one for educational purposes—any more than a statement that a

27

footballer has been 'injured' in a match is a useful predictor of his subsequent career as a player. In each case, there are a multitude of possibilities, many of which require more diagnostic information before a firm prognosis can be given.

At a more general level, too little attention has been paid to the environmentally determined, bio-social concomitants of retarded performance both of children living in very poor home circumstances, and of children in some forms of institutional care. The literature on the bio-medical effects of extreme poverty in the United States has recently been reviewed by Birch and Gussow (1970) in an impressive but disturbing volume concerned with health and welfare of the very poor. Many institutional children in United States institutions fare at least as badly as do children living in ghettoes—as Blatt (1967, 1969) among others has shown only too clearly. To expect short-term enrichment programmes to accomplish much while the material environment remains so poor is naïve.

A further weakness of compensatory studies has to do with the assumption that they can be concentrated solely on children in the pre-school years. Admittedly, the period of early childhood is a formative one, but there is now a wealth of evidence that aims achieved in compensatory programmes do not stick once children enter primary schooling. Instead, children tend to 'regress' educationally and intellectually to the level of control groups. The inference is plain: as Eisenberg and Conners (1968) have put it, 'we would not, after all, anticipate that a good diet at age five would protect a child against malnutrition at age six. The mind, like the brain, requires alimentation—bio-chemical, physiological, and cognitive—at every stage of its development [p. 122].' (See also a detailed and closely argued treatment of the same theme by Clarke, 1968.)

It should have come as no surprise to have discovered that, as Clarke (p. 1074) puts it, 'early learning will fade if not reinforced'. Gordon, in 1923, had reported a steady deterioration in IQ with age of canal-boat children who received irregular schooling. And Vernon (1957) in a longitudinal study, involving 865 boys aged fourteen years who had all been tested three years earlier before entering various types of secondary school, had shown the same phenomenon. In Vernon's study, after allowing for differences in initial ability of those entering different types of school, it was found that the mean IQ difference between boys in the 'best' school and those in the 'poorest' was 12·4 points. Similar findings, this time with young adults entering the Swedish army, were obtained by Husén (1951); and comparable data have been found when much older people have been tested.

Finally, a much more radical critique of compensatory education can be offered. As Bernstein (1970) has argued cogently, the very term *compensatory education* is a misnomer:

> [It] serves to direct attention away from the internal organization and the educational context of the school, and focus our attention on the families and children. 'Compensatory education implies that something is lacking in the family, and so in the child. As a result, the children are unable to benefit from schools.
>
> It follows, then, that the school has to 'compensate' for the something which is missing in the family, and the children are looked at as deficit systems. If only the parents were interested in the goodies we offer, if only they were like middle-class parents, then we could do our job. Once the problem is seen even implicitly in this way, it becomes appropriate to coin the terms 'cultural deprivation', 'linguistic deprivation', and so on. And then these labels do their own sad work.
>
> If the children are labelled 'culturally deprived', then it follows that the parents are inadequate; the spontaneous realization of their culture, its images and symbolic representations, are of reduced value and significance. Teachers will have lower expectations of the children, which the children will undoubtedly fulfil. All that informs the child — that gives meaning and purpose to him outside the school — ceases to be valid or accorded significance and opportunity for enhancement within the school. He has to orient towards a different structure of meaning, whether it is in the form of reading books (*Janet and John*), in the form of language use and dialect, or in the patterns of social relationships.
>
> ... The very form our research takes tends to confirm the beliefs underlying the organization, transmission and evaluation of knowledge by the school. Research proceeds by assessing the criteria of attainment that schools hold, and then measures the competence of different social groups in reaching these criteria. We take one group of children who we know beforehand possess attributes favourable to school achievements, and a second group of children who we know beforehand lack these attributes. Then we evaluate one group in terms of what it *lacks* when compared with another. In this way, research unwittingly underscores the notion of *deficit* and confirms the *status quo* of given organization, transmission and, in particular, evaluation of knowledge.

Bernstein's critique of compensatory education is that it distracts attention from the deficiencies in the school itself and focuses upon deficiencies within the community, family and child. We should, he says, stop thinking in terms of compensatory education and consider instead, most seriously and systematically, the conditions and contexts of the educational environment. These observations apply with a special force to much of the educational and psychological research which has been carried out on institutional children. Psychologists in particular have largely ignored the conditions in which the children live. At its narrowest, this approach leads to programmes of 'behaviour modification', which are concerned only with the alteration of types of behaviour which are a nuisance, or otherwise unacceptable to staff. The value of operant techniques for therapeutic purposes can scarcely be denied: but in themselves they provide no adequate solution to problems of institutional upbringing.

## 'Deprivation' in residential care

Research on the personality development and behaviour of children brought up in residential care has, like the research mentioned above, for the most part concentrated on the children and devoted little attention to the environment in which they live. By implication, however, deprivation studies offer a critique of the institutional environment. Where they are unsatisfactory is in their lack of specificity, in their tendency to lump together all types of institutional care as though they conformed to a common standard.

Research on the effects of separation from the mother, or deprivation of mother love in early infancy, is too well known to require extensive review. The literature has been summarized by Bowlby (1951), and reassessed by many writers (e.g. O'Connor, 1956; Ainsworth, 1962).

Only that part of the evidence derived from what Bowlby referred to as 'direct' studies of children in institutions and foster homes will be discussed briefly here.

Summarizing the evidence at that date, Bowlby became convinced that prolonged deprivation of the young child of maternal care is very likely to have grave and far-reaching effects on his character. The effects could be seen (1) during the period of separation; (2) during the period immediately after restoration to maternal care; and (3) permanently. They included various kinds of behaviour disturbance and long-term effects, of which the most serious were an incapacity to make affectionate relationships, retarded development, and the formation of a psychopathic character. Bowlby's monograph set off a controversy in which psychologists, child psychiatrists, psycho-analysts, paediatricians, ethologists, cultural anthropologists and sociologists all played a part. Ainsworth (1962), reassessing the literature after a further ten years of research, discussed several major controversial issues: the distinction between maternal deprivation and maternal separation; problems of multiple mothering; the extent, diversity and specificity of the effects—including the problems of delinquency and psychopathy; the permanence or irreversibility of the damage; and whether the effects might result from environmental deprivation rather than maternal deprivation, as well as other minor matters. Like Bowlby, Ainsworth was impressed by the congruity of the evidence, but she found the problem of interpretation no longer as simple as it might have appeared ten years earlier.

Many of the studies of maternal deprivation have much in common with the studies of the effects of environment on intelligence, and, indeed, both problems have frequently been studied together. The 'direct' studies cited by Bowlby are concerned mainly with very young babies in institutions. Thus Bakwin (1942, 1949) described the listlessness of infants under six months in institutions, and their unresponsiveness to familiar stimuli, while the failure of such babies to smile at the sight of a human face was reported in a series of well-known studies by Spitz and Wolf (1946). Progressive deviations from the norms of development by infants in institutions were described by Gesell and Armatruda (1947). Durfee and Wolf (1933), comparing the development of babies in different institutions, and analysing their findings by the amount of maternal care received before admission, found no harmful effects below the age of three months, but thereafter, the longer the children remained in institutions, the more severe their psychiatric disturbance. Bowlby pointed out with some insight that abnormal responses by the young child which took the form of listlessness or apathy might be welcomed by staff in institutions, because the children were easy to manage, whereas children suffering from normal distress reactions are not. The whole problem of the reactions of children's separation from their mothers was earlier discussed by Burlingham and Freud (1942, 1943) in two small but remarkable books in which they reported on their experience in a residential nursery with pre-school children of working mothers.

As already mentioned, one of the striking features of many institutional studies is the failure to distinguish between the effects of different types of institutional environment. Thus, Durfee and Wolf studied 118 children, living in several institutions, but the conditions in each are apparently assumed to be the same. Similarly, Simonsen (1947), in a much-quoted Scandinavian study, compared a group of 113 children aged between 1 and 4 years and living in 12 different institutions, with a group of children who lived at home. The results are presented in a simple contrast between the two groups, and differences within the institution group are largely ignored. Even when environmental differences among institutions are invoked as explanatory variables, this is usually done in order to interpret differences between the results of one study and another, a procedure which is questionable because of the lack of adequate description of the environments. Thus, Bowlby explains the smaller decrements in developmental quotient among an institutional group of children reported on by Levy (1947), when compared to the institutional group in the famous comparative study by Spitz (1945) by the 'better psychological conditions in which they lived'. In fact, few details of these conditions are given.

The main value of many deprivation studies lies in the attention which they have caused to be directed to the kinds of staffing patterns in institutions which might counter the ill effects of separation. An early account is given in Buhler (1935) of a study involving two groups of two-year-old children, cared for in the same nursery. One group was given very little tenderness, though adequately cared for in other respects. The second group had a nurse assigned to each child. At the end of half a year, the first group was mentally and physically retarded as compared with the second. Burlingham and Freud (1943) found that when all the children in their nursery were cared for collectively by all members of staff, the children showed signs of retarded development. They accordingly decided to change the pattern of organization and responsibility. The large nursery group was sub-divided into six small family groups of about four children in each, with an attendant or 'mother' in more or less complete charge of each family. She alone bathed and dressed her group, was responsible for their clothes, and offered them protection against the mishaps of nursery life. The intimacy at bath-times and in other situations, which became possible under this system, produced a remarkable improvement in speech. All the children greatly enlarged their vocabularies, and many who were backward in speech at the beginning of the change quickly made up the arrears. Not dissimilar findings have been obtained by Rheingold (1956, 1960).

In pointing to the psychological needs of young children for attention and care by familiar adults, the nursery studies quoted above have undoubtedly had a salutary effect on nursery organization. Burlingham and Freud's work was particularly important —indeed, the reorganization of residential nurseries in Britain after the Second World War followed very closely the recommendations made by these writers on the basis of their wartime experiences. This happened because of their profound psychological understanding of children and because their recommendations were practical and based on experience.

It cannot be denied, however, that others who have written on the ill effects of institutional upbringing have overstated their case, and some have laid great stress on matters which, on the face of it, appear trivial. Bettelheim (1959), for example, emphasized the need for the same adult to be involved in waking the children in the mornings. Roudinesco and Appell (1951) claimed good results from regular but relatively brief psycho-therapy sessions, but seem to have ignored—or been powerless to alter—the staffing patterns of the nursery they practised in. Spitz, according to Pinneau (1955), misreported his data in a manner which is indefensible. Bowlby himself must bear some responsibility not only for the closing of many residential nurseries in England, but for the cutting-down of day-nursery provision for the children of working mothers— presumably on the grounds that this would keep the mothers at home. As Wootton (1959, 1962) has pointed out, what the deprivation studies have mainly done is to expose the deplorable conditions in many of our institutions and the indifference of many hospitals to childish sensibilities. Other writers, notably Yarrow (1961), have drawn attention to the difficulty of deciding what it is in an institutional environment which retards or fosters the development of children.

The few quasi-experimental studies of residential upbringing of mentally handicapped children which have been undertaken (e.g. by Tizard, 1964), have contrasted small units, in which highly qualified research staff have participated in adequate numbers and over comparatively short periods, with backward, understaffed traditional institutions which have been greatly in need of reform. While such comparisons have been useful, they barely touch the problem of what are the main factors which determine patterns of care; and the actual description of the patterns of care investigated is impressionistic rather than systematic.

In short, in nearly all the research which has focused on the development of children in residential care, there has been relatively little attempt to characterize the child's environment, except in rather general terms. This is true of the classical studies mentioned above, and equally true of the many more recent studies listed by Dinnage and Pringle (1967) in their invaluable review of research in the United States, Western Europe, Israel and Great Britain between 1948 and 1966. 'Considering the volume of research over the past 18 years,' they say, 'it is disappointing that not more is known ... Most studies have been on too limited a scale and conducted over too short a period of time. Hence, only very limited generalizations are justified at this stage.' Dinnage and Pringle present an overview of the 'facts and fallacies' regarding residential care. They conclude that there are many questions for which there is, at present, insufficient evidence on which to base policy and practice. Significantly, they list 'institutional effects' among the questions about which least is known. They note that the majority of investigations have consisted of intensive case studies of relatively few children, and that the paucity of well-conducted studies is particularly marked in this area.

# 4 The sociology of residential institutions

Few of the studies of children in residential care reviewed in the last chapter have included a systematic account of the day-to-day environment of the child, or have discussed the way in which residential institutions actually function, or how function is related to structure. The sociology of residential organizations—a branch of organizational sociology still very much in its infancy—is concerned with these matters.

There have been several definitions of complex or formal organizations by different writers. While most of them agree on the essential ingredients of organizations, few have been successful in defining the extent of the field in strictly theoretical terms. Thus, James March (1965), writing the introduction to the most comprehensive reference book on organizations, was forced to describe the sociology of organizations as follows: 'It is what it is; and what it is can best be described by reading the detailed chapters.' There seems little point in contributing further general definitions of organizations in a monograph of this kind. Some complex organizations, however, as Parsons (1960) has pointed out, can be distinguished from others by the fact that they take the customer *into* the organization. In these organizations, 'the recipient of the service becomes an operative member of the service providing organization' (Parsons, 1960, p. 25). Residential institutions, as we understand them here, are characterized by this feature, and constitute a distinctive sub-type of complex organizations.

Until recently, most of the theoretical discussion and empirical research on the sociology of organizations have been in the areas of industrial sociology and public administration.* Only since the 1950s have prisons, churches, universities, hospitals, military establishments and other organizations occupied an important place in this field.

With the expansion of the field of the sociology of organizations have come many attempts to provide typologies. Among the best known are those by Blau and Scott (1963) and Etzioni (1961). Blau and Scott adopt a single criterion of who benefits from the operation of organizations (*cui bono*) as a means of classifying them; while Etzioni combines two variables, the kind of power applied to organization participants and the kind of involvement which participants have in the organization, to construct a typology based on what he calls the compliance relationship. All classificatory schemes have to be judged by their usefulness and both of these have proved extremely fruitful for some purposes. The former has been particularly helpful in identifying the central problem areas with which organizations of the different types have to deal: the latter has systematically pointed to the relationship between structural variables and motivational variables in organizations. Hall, Haas and Johnson (1967) have demonstrated, however, that neither typology differentiates clearly between organizations when a number of structural characteristics, such as complexity and degree of formalization, are examined. It is also the case that neither classification draws attention to the unique features of residential institutions, nor do they deal with the common problems encountered by such organizations. It is thus possible to locate examples of residential organizations in different sectors of both the Blau and Scott and the Etzioni classifications.

Although Parsons had drawn attention to the possible differences between residential organizations and other types, it was left to the distinguished American sociologist, Erving Goffman, to identify the boundaries of this organizational form and to describe its main attributes. Goffman (1961) pointed out—in a penetrating essay first published in 1957—that there was a fundamental difference between an organization which is devoted to the pursuit of war, to making money, to religious propaganda or to public administration, and one which has as its purpose the task of caring for persons who are in some sense dependent and who are taken into residence. At the same time, he observed that longstay residential

---

* Investigations describing non-industrial and non-governmental organizations have appeared in the literature from time to time – but these have tended to stand alone as isolated classics, unrepeated and unintegrated. Donald Clemmer's study *The Prison Community* (1940) is a case in point. It remained the only major sociological work on prisons until 1958, when *The Society of Captives* by Gresham Sykes was published.

institutions, irrespective of the purposes for which they were established, or of the category of persons whom they dealt with as inmates, tended to share certain characteristics. In this way, he delineated a field of study which would include all organizations which are expected to function as a more or less permanent, and more or less adequate, substitute home for a group of inmates who are cared for by a group of staff: that is, 'institutions' in the popular, non-sociological meaning of the term. We shall return briefly to the contribution of Goffman at the end of this chapter, but for the present we shall be concerned with the research that has taken place in residential institutions.

A striking feature of the sociological research in residential organizations is that it has been concerned mainly with those for adults. Gross (1956) commented that the systematic study of the school organization is yet to be made, and despite recent contributions in this area there is still some pertinence in that comment.*

Several studies of institutions for delinquent children exist, of which those by Polsky et al. (1962, 1968) are probably the most significant, and a recent case study by Flint (1967) gives an account of changes which tóok place in an institution for deprived children in Canada. A somewhat similar study, with severely retarded children, was earlier carried out by Tizard (1962, 1964). There have been a number of other studies of aspects of institutional life for the retarded—Dentler and Mackler (1961), Esher (1962), and MacAndrew and Edgerton (1964)—although few have been concerned solely with children. More recently, Morris (1969) and Martin, Bone and Spain (1971), have presented national data on mental subnormality hospitals in England, but they too have not been concerned primarily with children.

On the literature on residential institutions for adults, the research conducted in mental hospitals is reasonably representative and contains much of the most interesting material. Moreover, mental hospitals most nearly resemble the kinds of institutions with which this study is concerned, and our review of work is confined to studies of them. Since there have been several recent and comprehensive reviews of the literature on mental hospitals (Freidson, 1963; Perrow, 1965; Zusman, 1966; Ullmann, 1967; Wing and Brown, 1970), we have concentrated on matters which

---

* Although there have been many studies in recent years (see, for example, Hargreaves, 1967; Lacey, 1966; Holly, 1965; Gooch and Pringle, 1967; Eggleston, 1967), few have employed a consistent organizational framework. As Swift and Aclund (1969) have pointed out, the gain from these works 'has lain in the extent to which educationalists have accepted the need to carry out research along these lines and their growing sophistication and ability to think of schools as organizations' (p. 38).

are directly relevant to our own field of enquiry. The relevance of the sociology of organizations to medical services has been thoroughly examined by Scott (1966) and by Susser (1968).

## Case studies of mental hospitals

There has been a remarkable lack of comparative research into aspects of the functioning of the mental hospital. The traditional approach has taken the form of the single case study, which, at best, can provide only a descriptive and analytical account of a particular institution. Most writers have regarded the mental hospital as a complex, on-going social system, and the studies by Stanton and Schwartz (1954), Belknap (1956) and Caudill (1958) are perhaps the best known. In these, an attempt is made to describe the functioning of the mental hospital more or less in its entirety, and Caudill even goes so far as to treat the hospital as though it were a self-contained 'small society'. Somewhat less comprehensive reports which employ substantially the same approach are those by Dunham and Weinberg (1960) and Salisbury (1962). Two lesser-known studies, by Barrabee (1951) and Arnason (1958), employ a more formalized scheme of analysis, largely on Parsonian lines (Parsons, 1951, 1957).

The 'social system' approach has typically been linked with ideas deriving from the 'human relations' school of industrial sociology, and both Etzioni (1960) and Perrow (1965) have discussed the affinity between the ideas of the human relations movement and the theory and practice of psycho-therapy in mental institutions. The human relations school gives prominence to the role of communications in promoting organizational effectiveness and maintaining the morale of participants.* Where communication is found to be faulty, changes in the organizational structure are usually advocated to overcome the difficulty. Some problems in mental hospitals are doubtless problems of communication, but others are not, and, as Etzioni (1960) has suggested, the number of situations in which increased communication is likely to be effective is limited. The concern with organizational structure and its effects, through the communication process, on the care and treatment of patients is evident in much of the work cited above, particularly that by Stanton and Schwartz, and Caudill. In the writings associated with 'milieu therapy' and the development of 'therapeutic communities', these ideas become even more prominent (see Jones, 1953, 1968; Cumming and Cumming, 1962; Greenblatt, Levinson and Williams, 1957; Hyde and Solomon, 1950; Green-

* Two excellent recent discussions are provided by Mayntz (1964) and Brown (1967).

blatt, York and Brown, 1955). Typically in these studies, a social investigator, usually an anthropologist, works in collaboration with a psychiatrist. The techniques used have been mainly anthropological, particular attention being focused on 'informal' aspects of the organization's functioning. Interpretation of the results has usually involved a combination of structural-functional analysis and psychiatric theory.

The shortcomings of the anthropological approach have been amusingly put by Adams (1968), himself an anthropologist and writing in another context:

> The ethnographical investigator works in what has been called the context of discovery. Ethnographers, unlike their closest social science relatives, are much more concerned with making propositions than with testing them. While psychology, sociology and economics have developed sophisticated methods to test hypotheses, anthropology traditionally has been the unkempt country cousin, manure footing it along with unmanageable data. The difference, however, is not that ethnographers have been without a methodology but that the methodology relevant to their investigations lies in the context of discovery; and to be charitable, methodology in this area is scarcely sophisticated in any science.

The same point is put more tersely by Freud: it is easier to interpret the present than to predict the future.

Other case studies of mental hospitals derive their theory as much from role theory and the theory of bureaucracy as from structural-functional analysis and social system theory. In these studies attention is focused on, for example, the system—or, more properly, systems—of authority which prevail in the mental hospital, and on the importance of such systems for the role performance of different status groups among the staff or for the behaviour of the patients. Much of this research is also carried out with the collaboration of psychiatrists, but rather more attention is likely to be given to the formal aspects or organization structure. Of course, dividing lines between studies of different types are necessarily somewhat arbitary, and some of the studies cited earlier, notably that by Belknap (1956), have been concerned with these matters. Other studies of this type are those reported by Henry (1954, 1957), Dinitz, Lefton and Pasamanick (1959), and to some extent those by Cumming and Cumming (1956, 1962).

It is difficult to summarize the contribution of the many case studies. As Rapoport (1960) has pointed out, case studies have shown, in a variety of ways, that the patients' relationship with the psychiatric staff is only one factor in a field of forces which may greatly affect the therapeutic situation. In particular, they have shown that there are many features in the social organization of the mental hospital which have an adverse effect on the treatment of patients. We learn, for example, from Belknap (1956), Greenblatt, York and Brown (1955), Dunham and Weinburg (1960) among others, that because of the lack of psychiatric staff and their social distance from the wards, power resides in the attendant or aide role group, who have the least favourable stereotype of the patients. These writers suggest that aides may use their power to order 'shock' treatment as a disciplinary measure, and that in general they may replace the therapeutic values of the hospital with custodial values. Again, we learn from Belknap (1956) and Cumming and Cumming (1956) that the business side of the hospital has more power than the medical side, and that the attitudes of the lowest level employees in the business hierarchy can, through their maladministration, lead to shortages in food, clothing, bedding and soap at ward level, which adversely affect the quality of patient care.

Apart from these general considerations which affect the régimes in mental hospitals, one has to search the literature for the details of day-to-day events. For the most part, the scattered references are impressionistic. A few examples from the work of Stanton and Schwartz (1954) may be cited as representative. They found that general care was adequate 'only in respect of barest minimal needs': 'food was served under conditions that would be forbidding indeed for most people': 'bathing and dressing were hurried and routinized': and 'grace, charm and comfort seemed out of place' in the hospital they studied (p. 53). Later, they report that patients are prohibited from entering the kitchen, that meal-times and bed-times are rigidly fixed, and that clothes are locked away in places to which patients have no access (pp. 125-36). Still later, it is noted that the ward routine at meal-times, bath-times and bed-times is reinforced by the placement of non-conformist patients into seclusion. These routines were lengthy procedures, which could take up to nine hours of the patients' day (pp. 251-4). Useful though these impressions are, Stanton and Schwartz make little attempt to define such terms as 'minimal needs' or 'routinized procedures' and there is little in the way of systematic measurement and assessment.

Other examples could be quoted, but perhaps enough has been said to indicate the fragmentary and unsystematic nature of the documentation in this area. As a result, there seems to be general agreement at an impressionistic level that the traditional hospital is over-regimented and barren, but there is no way of telling the precise ways in which the regimentation occurs, nor the extent to which it is found in different settings. It would be difficult, for example, on the evidence presented by Stanton and Schwartz, to know whether the hospital they studied was more routinized in its procedure than, say, that studied by Caudill or by the Cummings. Much the same problem applies throughout organizational sociology for, as Etzioni (1961) has complained, even where quantitative techniques have been used, different instruments have been devised, using different methods of data collection and analysis, so that comparative assessment by secondary analysis of case studies is necessarily speculative.

This difficulty, of course, derives from the case study method itself. Udy (1965) has distinguished between the case study and the comparative study as follows: a case study describes an organization in detail by analysing the configuration of its parts, while the comparative study seeks generalizations about something by studying several instances of it. Thus, the case study may provide valuable insights and hypotheses, but it cannot yield generalizations of wide applicability.

## Comparative studies

Of the comparative studies of mental hospitals, two series have been singled out for comment. The first is the Psychiatric Evaluation Project (P.E.P.) set up as part of the Veterans Administration in the United States after the Second World War, and directed by Richard L. Jenkins (Jenkins and Gurel, 1959; Jenkins 1961). Ullmann (1967), who provides a tightly written and discriminating review of the best mental hospital literature, summarizes the findings of the P.E.P. studies and extends them through some similar research of his own, using slightly modified procedures.

The concern of both the P.E.P. and Ullmann was with the *effectiveness* of mental hospital programmes. A major problem, therefore, was to find criteria of effectiveness which would make quantitative studies possible. The measures finally selected by Ullmann were, first, the percentage of men released within 274 days after admission and who remained in the community for at least 90 consecutive days ('first significant release'); and, second, the percentage of men with two or more years' continuous hospitalization ('long hospitalization'). Ullmann makes a brave case for using length of hospital stay as his principal criterion of effectiveness, because of the difficulty of providing an acceptable definition of mental health and hence of directly measuring successful treatment. A smaller British study, by Jones and Sidebotham (1962), takes a somewhat similar approach for similar reasons. However, as Wing and Brown (1970) point out, such criteria are simply unacceptable. For studies such as ours, which are concerned mainly with

41

chronically handicapped children, few of whom are ever likely to be discharged from residential care, they are also irrelevant. The problem of the direct assessment of the effectiveness of such institutions has to be faced.

The second set of studies, by Wing and Brown (1970), are in a class by themselves, both methodologically and in the rigour with which they were carried out. Their investigations were 'primarily concerned with the adverse effects on schizophrenic patients of a prolonged stay in three selected mental hospitals and with the ways in which these effects could be counteracted and prevented'. The work began in 1960, and their method of approach in some ways influenced our own. The approach was deliberately quantitative: and as they say in their preface, 'We should be very content if our work were thought merely to have contributed some "hard and obstinate facts" . . . to a subject where theories are all too easily elaborated but are rarely meant to be tested.' And elsewhere, 'Practically all the material in this book is presented in numerical form. Such indices stand for real and important characteristics of personal condition and social environment, and we would reject the suggestion that is sometimes made (fortunately rather rarely) that they are meaningless abstractions. We have deliberately chosen to make our investigation in this way because we do not think that the most animated and evocative description by the most perceptive participant observers could possibly answer the questions we set ourselves. We do not, of course, discount their value, but they have another purpose and are complementary to the present approach.'

What is particularly valuable methodologically about this work is the success which the investigators achieved in developing quantitative scales by which to measure the severity of schizophrenic patients' handicaps, and their skill in *measuring* the social poverty of the environment in which the patients lived. We have adapted some of the techniques developed by Wing and Brown for our own purposes, and these are referred to later in the text.

For Wing and Brown's investigations into institutionalism and schizophrenia, three hospitals were selected for study which seemed to differ markedly in social conditions and administrative policy. At each, a random sample of approximately 100 female schizophrenic patients who had been in hospital for more than two years and who were less than sixty years of age was selected. The diagnosis was checked from case notes and at interviews with the patients. In 1960, the investigators spent a week at each hospital, interviewing patients and staff and collecting information. Further surveys were carried out in two of the hospitals in 1962 and in all three hospitals in 1964 and 1967. The interest of the investigators lay in the nature of the associations between the clinical condition of the patients and the characteristics of the social environment in which they lived.

The clinical measures used by Wing and Brown need not concern us here: they were based on highly reliable assessments obtained from psychiatric interview, from case notes and from nurses' ratings of ward behaviour, and they included a rating scale on 'attitude to discharge' which was the main measure of institutionalism. The social conditions of the ward were also assessed in several ways, using different sources of information. Measures included: (1) an inventory of all the personal possessions of each patient in the series which was made after interviewing the patients and nursing staff, and checking with the patient the contents of lockers and wardrobes; (2) a 'time budget' in which information was collected about all activities from the time of getting up until going to bed — what time the patient rose, who woke her, whether she dressed herself and how long this took, the details of her toilet, whether she made her bed, how long she waited for breakfast, and so on through the day; (3) nurses' opinions about each patient's ability to cope with certain everyday activities and responsibilities; for example, whether she could visit the local shop without asking, whether she could do useful work in the hospital, or go out with a male patient; (4) the daily occupation, if any, of the patient; (5) contact with the outside world, including whether she went home, had town parole or ground parole, or was visited, and how often each of these occurred; (6) a thirty-five-item scale of ward restrictiveness which was filled in after questioning the nurses. The items were concerned with restrictions on the movement of patients, such as locking of ward doors, the necessity for staff permission to leave the ward, and so on, and with more general rules and routines — restrictions on the use of the bathroom, regulations about personal clothing, access to the ward kitchen, and so on.

In addition, other information about the patients and their social backgrounds, the drugs they were receiving and the clinical course of their illness was collected.

Brown and Wing were able to show that in each hospital there was close association between the patients' clinical condition and the social condition of the different wards in which they lived. These factors were in turn related to length of stay and to attitudes towards discharge. Thus, the original hypothesis that patients living in widely differing social environments would present different patterns of symptomatology was confirmed.

However, further questions remained: does the social environment influence the patient, or do the patients create their own environment? Were the patients in the three hospitals different in some way which was not caused by, but was rather the cause of, differences in the social environment in which they lived? Were longer-stay patients those who had *elected* to remain in hospital, and were these same patients those who made for themselves a socially unstimulating environment? The follow-up data answered these questions by providing information about all those patients in the original study who remained in the hospital over a seven-and-a-half-year period. This included the great majority. A striking association was shown, in each hospital, and for patients of different ages, length of stay and severity of clinical condition, between changes on all social measures of the patients' environment, and measures of clinical condition, especially social withdrawal. A most interesting finding was that, in general, there was an improvement in social conditions between 1960 and 1964 in all three hospitals, and a deterioration between 1964 and 1967. These changes in social conditions were paralleled by corresponding changes for the better and for the worse in the patients' clinical state. As the authors say:

> The various stages of this study point towards a conclusion which is very difficult to resist—that a substantial proportion, though by no means all, of the morbidity shown by longstay schizophrenic patients in mental hospitals is a product of their environment. The social pressures which acted to produce this morbidity can, to some extent, be counteracted, but the process of reform may itself have a natural history and an end ...The hypothesis that the social conditions under which the patient lives (particularly poverty of the social environment) are actually responsible for part of the symptomatology (particularly the negative symptoms), has been subjected to a number of fairly rigorous tests, any one of which it might well have failed, but it has not been disproved ... Not only can it be demonstrated that the social treatments carried out by mental hospital staff do have value and that the course of schizophrenic illnesses can be influenced in hospital, as it can outside, but there is a salutary reminder that efforts must be kept up and that reform itself has a natural history. This demonstration has lessons and a warning for social psychiatrists.

This series of studies, which was carried out about the same time as our own, has been described in some detail because it illustrates a method of approach which we ourselves have used, though in a somewhat different way. The essential methodological features include the use of multiple and independent indices of social and clinical condition, drawn from different sources and previously shown to be reliable and to have a 'construct' validity which makes them suitable for their purpose. In Wing and Brown's study, attention was focused on the one hand on different behavioural patterns which were regarded as aspects of the patients' clinical state, and on the other hand on different measures of the ward environment. In our studies, which were all cross-sectional, the primary centre of interest was in the ward environment. We have, however, attempted to relate differences in the ward environment—more specifically in 'child management practices' and staff-child interactions—to differences in the organizational structure of the institutions we studied; and in so far as our limited data permitted, we have tried to relate differences in the ward environment to the behaviour of the children. That some relationship would be found among these variables is perhaps hardly surprising: but the nature of the associations and the particular factors which systematically determine their strengths are by no means obvious. To show how the social organization of an institution influences the patterns of behaviour shown by the staff to the patients, and how these in turn affect the development and behaviour of children, are matters requiring detailed empirical study.

## Erving Goffman and the concept of the 'total institution'

Before leaving this brief overview of theory and research in residential organizations, we must return to the work of Goffman. We have already pointed to the contribution of Goffman in delineating residential institutions as an organizational form and establishing them as a field for sociological enquiry. He referred to them as *total institutions,* and he defined them denotatively by listing them in five rough groupings. First, there are institutions established to care for persons felt to be both incapable and harmless, such as homes for the blind, the aged, the orphaned and the indigent. Second, there are places which care for persons felt to be incapable and a threat to the community, however unintended: mental hospitals, T.B. sanitoria and leper colonies exemplify this group. Third, prisons, concentration camps and P.O.W. camps are total institutions designed to protect the community against what are felt to be intentional dangers to it. Fourth, there are institutions which pursue some work-like task, such as army barracks, ships, boarding schools, colonial camps and large mansions. Finally, there are establishments organized as retreats from the world, such as monasteries, abbeys, convents and other cloisters (Goffman, 1961, pp. 4-5).

Two basic features distinguish these total institutions from other social establishments, according to Goffman: their 'encompassing or total character' (p. 4) and the fact that 'the staff [in] their work, and hence their world, have uniquely to do with people. This people-work is not quite like personnel work or the work of those involved in service relationships; the staff, after all, have objects and products to work upon, not services, but these objects and products are people' (p. 74). Because of these features, says Goffman, the total institution is a social hybrid, part residential community, part formal organization; therein lies its special sociological interest.

Goffman goes on to give an account of the characteristics of such institutions and of the staff and inmate 'worlds', which is both powerful and compelling. In everyday life, he points out, individuals tend to sleep, play and work in different places, with different co-participants, under different authorities, and without an overall, rational plan. On the other hand, 'the central feature of total institutions may be described as a breakdown of the barriers ordinarily separating these three spheres of life. First, all aspects of life are conducted in the same place and under the same single authority. Second, each phase of the members' daily activity is carried out in the immediate company of a large batch of others, all of whom are treated alike and required to do the same thing together. Third, all phases of the days' activities are tightly scheduled, with one activity leading at a prearranged time into the next, the whole sequence of activities being imposed from above by a system of explicit formal rulings and a body of officials. Finally, the various enforced activities are brought together into a single rational plan, designed to fulfil the official aims of the institution' (p. 6).

Goffman's account is not based on direct empirical study of particular establishments; rather it draws upon a wealth of examples culled from literature—fictional and biographical as well as sociological—to illustrate the points he makes. It is, for the sociology of institutions, what *War and Peace* is for military science —a brilliant and unforgettable classic which describes the most poignant aspects of the subject.

We were ourselves much influenced by Goffman, but found his ideas difficult to use in empirical research. For although he shows in a graphic way that similarities may exist between what hitherto had been regarded as quite disparate institutions, he does so by the use of an *ideal type* construct which does not have the flexibility required for comparative and empirical investigations. In his assumption that the features he describes correlate in a consistent and coherent pattern, Goffman makes of the total institution a single unitary type, marked off from other organizations both qualitatively and quantitatively by discontinuities from those next in line. With Goffman's concept as it stands, one is presented with the problem that when looking at any particular institution, one can say little more than it is, or is not, total—according to how well it conforms to the ideal type. But what if some institutions are more total than others? What if an institution has only some of the features which are said to characterize the total institution? Which, if any, of the characteristics of a total institution are the central ones?

For some time it has been recognized in psychology that such complex qualities as intelligence and personality, each of which may contain a number of variables or dimensions, vary continuously throughout the general population. The discontinuities of the kind presumed to exist by classical writers using conventional 'type' concepts—for example, in personality research or studies of physique—rarely exist in nature (Eysenck, 1960).

In recent years, sociologists too have been moving towards similar conclusions: thus Udy (1959), Hall (1963a, b), Pugh *et al.* (1963) have come to question whether the constituent elements of Weber's (1957) ideal type of bureaucracy, for example, are in fact interrelated in the way he assumed. This has led them to suggest alternative formulations in terms of continuous variables, the relationships between which are seen as problematic. It seems unlikely also that the kinds of discontinuities postulated by Goffman in the field of residential institutions will be found in practice.

We therefore abandoned the unitary concept of total institutions, and, using some of Goffman's ideas and terminology as a starting point, moved towards operational definitions of conceptually distinct elements and their measurement. The relations between these elements were treated as matters for empirical study. Our approach has thus been piecemeal and analytical as opposed to holistic. We have devised a scale to measure one important dimension of residential organizations—inmate management—and applied it in institutions for children. We have related the findings on this dimension to some organizational features of the institutions we have studied. In the long run, however, the development of other scales to measure various attributes of residential institutions should permit the taking of a dimensional approach to the problem of classification in this field. What we have done, we think, has been to make a beginning in this direction.

**part two**

**Varieties of residential care:
Field studies**

# 5  Four large institutions

As has been mentioned in Chapter 1, it is clear from observation that, at least in contemporary England, the manner in which children are brought up in longstay hospitals is very different from the manner in which 'deprived' children who do not present mental or physical handicaps are brought up in modern, longstay children's homes. However, few detailed studies of such homes and hospitals have been undertaken and our first investigations— which were descriptive and analytical—focus on the daily life of children in different types of residential care. Four large longstay institutions were selected for the first study. Two of these were homes for children 'in care'; that is, children who required substitute care for family reasons, either because they had no parents or because their parents were unable to care for them at home. The other two institutions were children's hospitals. One was a large paediatric hospital which included a number of wards for longstay cases, and the other was a mental subnormality hospital which cared only for severely retarded children.

The aims of the study were four-fold: first, to describe the manner in which children were brought up in these contrasting institutions; second, to describe the organization of the establishments in which the children were cared for; third, to develop quantitative techniques for measuring aspects of the children's environment; and fourth, to develop hypotheses which could subsequently be tested about factors which might account for any observed differences in the patterns of residential care.

Preliminary fieldwork in the four institutions began late in 1963. The two sociologists spent more than eight months observing staff and children in seventy-nine separate units in which children lived. Three series of standardized interviews were carried out, with appropriate grades of staff. The interviews were designed to elicit information about the handicaps and abilities of the children; the routine activities of the children; and the organization of the establishments and the personal histories of the staff. Further information was collected by examining case records, standing orders, off-duty sheets, pay sheets and other documents. Check lists were used to record the existence of various facilities. The data are presented in this and the following two chapters.

## The four establishments

Before describing the institutions, we must first say a few words by way of definition. Throughout this monograph we use the terms 'institution' and 'establishment' interchangeably. We have not found it necessary to provide a rigorous definition of the term institution, but we have used it in what we take to be its common-sense meaning: that is, to describe a building or set of buildings, together with its residents and staff, which occupies an identifiably separate site and serves some more or less explicit and identifiable purpose. In deciding just what constitutes the residential institution, the major complicating factor is the probability that the responsibilities of a particular person or group of persons may extend beyond the physical boundaries of location to include several different organizational sites. This situation makes it possible to define a 'hospital', for example, in several different ways. Thus the *Hospitals Year Book* for 1966 lists subnormality hospitals as one institution if they come under the same *Hospital Management Committee*. On the other hand, Morris (1969), in her recent survey, defines a hospital 'as a group of patients and staff, *whether housed together in a single complex or not,* under the charge of a single *Medical Superintendent*'.* In the present studies, any group of patients occupying a separate site, or cared for by a separate staff, has been treated as though it constituted a separate hospital, *regardless* of whether it was grouped with others under the same Medical Superintendent or the same management committee. We have taken a similar approach where other organizations occupy several sites.

Each definition has its limitations. With our definition, it could be argued that we run the risk of over-simplifying organizational structure and of excluding the organizational problems of central-peripheral relations from consideration. In practice, these problems have been greatly diminished by the fact that, in all cases reported in this monograph, we have studied the establishment from which

---

* Morris (1969), p. 28. Emphasis added.

the chief executive administers the organization, and, so long as the problem of peripheral units is borne in mind, we see no difficulty in taking them into account where this is appropriate.

In the sense referred to above, the four institutions were about the same size, at least in terms of the number of residents. The first home had 340 children, the second 377, the subnormality hospital 307 and the paediatric hospital 368. Both the children's homes were grouped cottage homes, administered by the children's department of the Local Authority in their area. Each occupied its own distinctive site and neither organization had any peripheral units. The two hospitals, on the other hand, formed part of the same hospital group and were administered by the same hospital management committee, appointed by the Regional Hospital Board under the National Health Service. The two hospitals shared a common location, although they occupied separate parts of the site and employed separate medical and nursing staffs.

The first home consists of a single estate of detached houses set along both sides of a tree-lined avenue. A short drive joins the avenue at right-angles and leads to the nearby main road. The whole site is enclosed by a wooden fence about five feet high. The main road leads quickly to suburban areas of population on the far outskirts of London, but socially the estate forms no part of the surrounding neighbourhood.

The administrative block—known as 'Staff House'—and the house of the Superintendent are situated at the intersection of drive and avenue. The separation from the local community is balanced by the provision of community facilities within the establishment. At various points along the main avenue can be found a church, a primary school, a nursery school, a library, a sick bay, a remedial education unit, a small swimming pool and three 'shops'. There are also houses for the deputy superintendent and the chief engineer, an annexe for other staff, several outhouses and a small lodge by the main entrance. At one end of the avenue is the gymnasium, which is used as an activities centre, and at the other end are the playing fields. Between Staff House and the gymnasium on one side, and between Staff House and the playing fields on the other, are the houses in which the children are accommodated.

The second home occupies a much larger site, but, physically at least, it is more closely integrated into the surrounding community. Like the first home, it consists of a number of houses grouped together in the form of a single estate, the whole site being circumscribed by a fence. But in this case, one of the two avenues which make up the estate joins a suburban street. On one side there are shops and on the other are private residences. Buses stop outside the entrance, and there is no sense of physical isolation and remoteness.

The main avenue runs in a more or less straight line from the front entrance to the back entrance of the establishment. A second avenue forms a large, U-shaped loop which meets the main avenue at two points. The houses which provide the accommodation for the children are situated along both these avenues.

Substantially similar community buildings are provided at the second home as those already described for the first; an administration block, a staff centre, a community centre, sick bay, nursery school, clothing store, shoe store, food store and a swimming pool are all to be found within the grounds. Houses are provided for the Superintendent and his deputy as well as for the engineer. One of the major differences at this level of provision is that the second home has its own laundry on the site.

The two hospitals are situated in a suburban area very like that of the second home. The extensive grounds are surrounded by fences and hedges, and access to the hospital is gained by following a long, residential street which leads from the railway station just over a mile distant. The hospitals arrange transport for visitors at certain times, and it is not unusual to find a hospital bus outside the station to meet passengers.

A curving drive leads to a large administrative block, behind which are the main hospital grounds. The site is divided by a straight central avenue, and three parallel streets branch off from each side of the avenue. The narrow streets are separated from each other by expanses of well-kept lawn and shrubbery. It is along these side-streets that the hospital wards are situated. For the most part, the wards of the paediatric hospital are to the left of the avenue, while the wards of the subnormality hospital are to the right. A few streets, however, have wards from both hospitals.

A school for the children in the subnormality hospital is situated at the far end of the central avenue, and this occupies the ground floor of an old two-storey building. On the first floor, the nurse training schools are accommodated and these provide separate tuition for student nurses in both hospitals. Two wards have been converted for use as schoolrooms for those children in the paediatric hospital who are able to get up to attend school. Playing fields, a small zoo, a recreation hall and a chapel complete the facilities available for the children. The zoo is intended primarily for the use of children in the subnormality hospital and the recreation hall is used mainly by the children in the paediatric hospital.

A number of specialist departments offer facilities to both hospitals: X-ray, physiotherapy, speech therapy, psychology, pharmacy, pathology, social service and so on. Some of these departments are housed in the main administration block, while others occupy converted wards no longer required for patients. A large laundry, just to the left of the administrative block, serves both hospitals as well as other nearby hospitals. At the eastern end of the site, sports fields, tennis courts and a club-house provide recreational facilities for the staff of both hospitals. Many of the nursing staff are accommodated in a large nurses' home, and there is also a house for the medical administrator, close to the main entrance.

The paediatric hospital has no outlying units on other sites, although it runs its own out-patients service. There are, however, a number of other subnormality units which are part of the same hospital group. Five small units, some close by and others further away, together provide a further 200 beds. Another large hospital has recently been added to the group which could potentially provide accommodation for 700 adult subnormal patients, although at the time of our research it housed just over 400. The responsibility for the smaller units is shared between the consultants and matrons of the two large subnormality hospitals.

## The living units

We use the term 'living unit' to describe the smallest unit of accommodation, the day-to-day functioning of which is the formally delegated responsibility of one or more senior members of staff. Thus the basic living units in the children's homes are houses under the responsibility of housemothers, while those in the two hospitals are wards, under the care of sisters or charge nurses. This usage differs from that of Morris (1969), who appears to use the term synonymously with the way in which we have defined 'institution' above.*

The living units in both of the children's homes were known to staff and children as 'cottages', and each cottage was identified by the name of a tree or plant. The first home had twenty-three cottages, one of which was used to accommodate households whose own cottage was under decoration or repair, so that only twenty-two units were in use at any one time. Some cottages were designed to hold up to fifteen children, others up to twenty children. The smaller cottages contained a staff sittingroom, a kitchen, a general livingroom, a bathroom and a lavatory on the ground floor,

---

* See Morris (1969), p. 77. In her study, Morris describes several sites under the same Medical Superintendent as 'a hospital', while each of the separate sites constitutes 'a living unit'. A living unit, in Morris's sense of the term, may thus consist of a number – in some cases a large number – of physically separate wards.

while the larger ones had an extra sittingroom—usually used as a diningroom—and an extra bathroom and storage room. All cottages had bedrooms for staff and children upstairs as well as additional bathing and toilet facilities. Just over half the children, 52·5 per cent, slept in bedrooms containing five beds, while more than one-fifth, 22·8 per cent, had single rooms or shared with one other child. In the second home, thirty of the thirty-six cottages were semi-detached; the remaining six were detached and these were the only buildings in any of the four institutions to have been built since the Second World War. All cottages were designed to hold up to twelve children and had substantially similar accommodation. This consisted of a livingroom, diningroom, kitchen and two 'bowl' rooms containing wash basins and w.c.s on the ground floor, and bedrooms for staff and children, bathrooms, toilets and storage facilities on the first floor. The detached cottages had an extra playroom and cloakroom downstairs and an additional bathroom upstairs. No children were in bedrooms with more than four beds; less than half, 47·7 per cent, were in three-bedded rooms, and 21·2 per cent had single rooms or shared with one other child. Nearly all of the cottages in both homes had extra toilet facilities for children playing outside. Only the six newer cottages in the second home had central heating.

The living units in both hospitals were known to staff and children alike as 'wards', and each ward was identified by a letter and a number. All of the wards in the hospitals were semi-detached, single-storey buildings, built to basically the same design. Internal modifications had been carried out in the subnormality wards, however, which distinguished them from those in the paediatric hospital. The subnormality hospital had sixteen units, most of which tended to specialize in the care of children with particular grades of mental defect. Each ward was designed to care for twenty patients, and the accommodation consisted of one dayroom, one dormitory, a kitchen, an office, a treatment room and an annexe containing baths and toilets. Most wards had a small cubicle which could be used for isolation purposes, but which was usually used for storage. Each semi-detached pair of wards shared a fenced courtyard at the rear. All of the children normally slept in dormitory accommodation. The paediatric hospital had sixteen shortstay wards—three acute surgical, one general surgical, three orthopaedic, two E.N.T. and seven acute medical—and seven long-stay wards—two medical, two muscular dystrophy, one cerebral palsy, one poliomyelitis and one psychiatric. Internally, the long-stay wards were similar to the units in the subnormality hospital and all of the children in them slept in dormitories. Shortstay wards, however, had two dormitories and no dayroom. The second dormitory was subdivided into a number of isolation cubicles. Wards in the paediatric hospital had courtyards similar to those in the subnormality hospital. None of the wards in either hospital had outside toilet facilities. All of the wards in both hospitals were centrally heated.

Since our main interest was in the long-term care of children in institutions, it was decided to limit the study in the paediatric hospital to the longstay wards. In the event, it was not possible, for administrative reasons, to study one of the medical wards for girls or the psychiatric ward, and only the five remaining wards, which were the responsibility of the same consultant, were included. All the figures in the text and tables, therefore, refer to these five wards in the paediatric hospital. We studied all the living units in the other three institutions.

Table 5.1 summarizes the details of the size of living units for the four institutions. The largest units were those in the subnormality hospital; the smallest those in the second home. The units in the first home and in the paediatric hospital were of very similar size. In no case could the living units be described as large or overcrowded.

TABLE 5.1   *Size of living units in four establishments and percentages of children living in units of different sizes*

| | No. children | No. units | Mean size | % children in units with less than 10 children | % children in units 10–14 children | % children in units 15 or more children |
|---|---|---|---|---|---|---|
| First home | 340 | 22 | 15·5 | 2·6 | 7·8 | 89·4 |
| Second home | 377 | 36 | 10·5 | 9·3 | 91·7 | 0·0 |
| S.S.N. hospital | 307 | 16 | 19·2 | 0·0 | 0·0 | 100·0 |
| Paediatric hospital[a] | 83 | 5 | 16·6 | 0·0 | 15·7 | 84·3 |

[a]In this table, as in subsequent references, the figures for the paediatric hospital relate solely to the five long-stay wards.

While none of the cottages in either home was luxuriously furnished, all were able to provide a reasonable standard of comfort. There were, for example, enough easy chairs for the

57

residents to sit down together if they wanted to, and most rooms had carpets or rugs on the floors. Some cottages could have benefited from redecoration, but without exception they had a clean and 'lived in' appearance. Most of the cottages in both homes had been successful in avoiding an institutional atmosphere by varying the patterns of curtains, bedspreads, wallpapers and so on from room to room. All of the children had some private space in which to keep their possessions—some had drawers, others lockers—although no housemother in either home felt that these facilities were entirely adequate. The second home in particular was extremely lacking in hanging-space for clothes to which the children had direct access. All cottages had a television set, though these were not provided by the Local Authority: usually, staff and children contributed to the rental.

The wards in both hospitals were well furnished by hospital standards, although six of the wards in the subnormality hospital were badly in need of redecoration. In contrast to the cottages in the homes, however, they lacked warmth and homeliness. None of the wards had carpets and only two wards in the paediatric hospital and none in the subnormality hospital had any easy chairs for patients or staff. All of the wards except one in the subnormality hospital had a locker for each child, although for the most part these were used to store bed-linen rather than personal possessions. All children in the paediatric hospital had bedside lockers. There were very few wardrobes in either hospital, and most clothes were stored centrally. All units had television sets provided by the establishments. Beds in the dormitories of both hospitals were lined along each wall, and the physical layout, furnishing and decoration were virtually identical from ward to ward. The physical conditions in the subnormality hospital, however, were very much better than those generally reported by Morris (1969)—the distance between beds was more than three feet in most wards and the buildings were light, airy and free from offensive smells.

The availability of bathing, washing and toilet facilities for the four establishments are summarized in Table 5.2. It can be seen that the two homes were better provided with baths and wash basins than the two hospitals; the second home, on average, was twice as well provided, and the first home one-and-a-half times as well provided, as the hospitals in these respects. The differences between the institutions in the provision of toilets, however, were much smaller, and the first home was indeed worse off than the hospitals in this matter.

Once again, it is interesting to note that the subnormality hospital

TABLE 5.2 *Ratios of bathing, washing and toileting facilities to children in four establishments*

| Facility | Institution | Total units | Total Residents | Mean Ratio | Ratio better than 1-5 children | | Ratio better than 1-10 children | | Ratio worse than 1-10 children | |
|---|---|---|---|---|---|---|---|---|---|---|
| | | | | | No. units | % Residents | No. units | % Residents | No. units | % Residents |
| Baths | 1st home | 22 | 340 | 1:7·7 | 1 | 3 | 21 | 97 | 0 | 0 |
| | 2nd home | 36 | 377 | 1:5·7 | 15 | 40 | 21 | 60 | 0 | 0 |
| | Paediatric | 5 | 83 | 1:12·0 | 0 | 0 | 2 | 41 | 3 | 59 |
| | S.S.N. | 16 | 307 | 1:9·9 | 0 | 0 | 15 | 93 | 1 | 7 |
| Wash basins | 1st home | 22 | 340 | 1:3·6 | 18 | 80 | 4 | 20 | 0 | 0 |
| | 2nd home | 36 | 377 | 1:2·5 | 36 | 100 | 0 | 0 | 0 | 0 |
| | Paediatric | 5 | 83 | 1:4·9 | 3 | 57 | 2 | 43 | 0 | 0 |
| | S.S.N. | 16 | 307 | 1:5·3 | 10 | 62 | 5 | 31 | 1 | 7 |
| W.c.s.[a] | 1st home | 22 | 340 | 1:10·3 | 0 | 0 | 12 | 57 | 10 | 43 |
| | 2nd home | 36 | 377 | 1:5·3 | 23 | 62 | 13 | 38 | 0 | 0 |
| | Paediatric | 5 | 83 | 1:6·3 | 2 | 41 | 0 | 0 | 3 | 59 |
| | S.S.N. | 16 | 307 | 1:4·9 | 9 | 56 | 4 | 25 | 3 | 19 |

[a] All cottages in the first home and 22 cottages in the second home had one or more outside W.c.s. Some cottages used these as additional storage space, and for the most part the children used these facilities only when they were playing outside. Moreover, at certain times, during the night, the staff toilet was available to the children, in several cottages.

studied here enjoyed better toilet and washing facilities than those generally reported by Morris (1969).*

## The children

In each establishment there were proportionately more boys than girls: 55 per cent were boys in the first home, 62 per cent in the second, 60 per cent in the subnormality hospital and 69 per cent in the paediatric hospital. For the most part, units in all establishments were for both sexes, although there was one unit in the first home for boys only, and five similar units in the second home. In the subnormality hospital there were five wards for boys and one for girls, and there were two wards for boys in the paediatric hospital.

Each establishment also had proportionately more longstay residents—defined as two months or longer—than shortstay cases: 88 per cent were longstay in the first home, 93 per cent in the second, 98 per cent in the subnormality hospital and 100 per cent in the paediatric hospital.† In fact, the majority of children in all the living units we studied would remain there for years rather than months.

The populations in all four establishments were also roughly comparable in terms of their age composition:

TABLE 5.3  *Percentage distribution of children by age categories in four establishments*

|  | No. children | Birth to 4 years | 5–10 years | 11–14 years | 15 years or over |
|---|---|---|---|---|---|
| First home | 340 | 10·0 | 42·6 | 39·4 | 7·9 |
| Second home | 377 | 14·4 | 48·8 | 32·4 | 4·5 |
| S.S.N. | 307 | 11·0 | 54·3 | 34·7 | 0·0 |
| Paediatric | 83 | 16·9 | 36·1 | 21·7 | 25·3 |

The two children's homes were not significantly different from each other in terms of age composition of the children in them. The subnormality hospital differed from the other three establish-

* According to Morris (1969), p. 94, more than 50 per cent of the patients in her hospital sample were in units with ratios of one w.c. to seven or more patients, and 19 per cent in units with a ratio of one to ten or more; 64·2 per cent were in units where more than fifteen patients shared a bath, and 1·2 per cent where there were no baths at all. Morris gives no figures for the ratio of wash basins to patients.
† In the paediatric hospital we had, of course, excluded shortstay wards: the hospital as a whole provided 126 beds for longstay cases and 319 for shortstay cases, giving a total capacity of 445 beds. Only 368 of the beds were filled at the time of our survey.

ments in having no children over the age of fourteen years in residence. By this age, subnormal children were transferred to a sister hospital within the group. The paediatric hospital had a slightly higher proportion of children under the age of five and a markedly higher proportion over the age of fourteen, with correspondingly lower proportions in the middle age groups. The older children in the paediatric hospital were all resident in two wards which cared for youths suffering from muscular dystrophy. The remaining three wards closely resembled the living units in the other three institutions as far as age composition was concerned.

The children in the four establishments were very different in terms of mental ability and physical handicap. Those in the two homes were mostly of normal intelligence. Records of intelligence tests were not available in the homes and we made no special study of this. However, all the children were receiving full-time education or were in full-time employment. Table 5.4 shows the proportions attending different types of school.

TABLE 5.4  *Percentage distribution of children by type of schooling in the two children's homes*

|  | No. children | Nursery schools | Primary schools | Secondary schools | Full-time work |
|---|---|---|---|---|---|
| First home | 340 | 8·8 | 47·9 | 41·5 | 1·8 |
| Second home | 377 | 12·5 | 52·8 | 34·5 | 0·3 |

The educational provision for all children in the homes was by the Local Education Authority, and in both cases a primary and a nursery school were provided in the grounds of the establishment. Children over the age of eleven went outside to Local Authority secondary schools, which were attended also by other children living in their own homes. These schools were often at a considerable distance from the institutions and it was a deliberate policy of the children's departments to have the children attending many separate schools, so that the concentration of deprived children was not too high in any one school. Children from the first home went to thirty-four separate secondary schools, no school having more than thirteen children from the establishment. Children from the second home went to twenty-two separate secondary schools, with a maximum of twenty-three children from the establishment attending the same school. Twenty children from the first home attended special schools, including fifteen who went to a remedial education unit within the establishment. Five children from the second home attended special schools. Most of the children attending special schools were educationally subnormal.

Few children in either of the homes had physical handicaps of moderate or severe degree. All of them were fully ambulant. There were no children, other than infants, who were unable to speak at all, and although some children were backward in their speech, communication was not a serious problem. Similarly, all of the children apart from the youngest were able to feed, dress and wash themselves without assistance. Incontinence was a problem in some cottages, though rarely such a problem as was found in the hospitals: 13 per cent of the children in the first home and 15 per cent in the second wet their beds or pants at least once in a week.

It was evident, however, that many of the children manifested symptoms of maladjustment and neurotic disorder. Data were collected about the behaviour of children in the homes using the Child Behaviour Scales developed by Rutter (1967). These scales were designed as screening devices to pick out deviant children. There are two forms: Scale A completed by parents, and Scale B completed by teachers. In the present study, housemothers were asked to complete the forms normally filled in by parents. A child scoring thirteen or more on Scale A, or nine or more on Scale B, is considered to be deviant. In the first home, 38 per cent of the boys and 23 per cent of the girls had scores of thirteen or more on Scale A; in the second home the proportions were 23 per cent of the boys and 22 per cent of the girls. The differences between the two homes in the proportions of deviant boys are greatly reduced when the teachers' ratings, using Scale B, are compared: 41 per cent of boys and 29 per cent of girls in the first home, and 35 per cent of boys and 28 per cent of girls in the second home, had deviant scores of nine or more.*

Recent data, from a study on the Isle of Wight (Rutter, Tizard and Whitmore, 1970), where Scales A and B were completed for 3,200 children aged ten to twelve years, suggest that about 7·4 per cent of boys and 5·4 per cent of girls can be expected to receive deviant scores on Scale A, while 9·8 per cent of boys and 4·8 per cent of girls score deviantly on Scale B. The proportions of both boys and girls in both the homes, therefore, are several times higher than would have been expected in a population of children living in their own homes. There are several reasons, however, why these data should be interpreted with some caution: houseparents, rather than natural parents, were asked to complete Scale

* We are indebted to our colleague, William Yule, for the analysis and interpretation of the Behaviour Scale data.

A, and their professional training and experience may have influenced scores; the children were known to be in the care of Local Authorities and there may have been a greater readiness to attribute behaviour problems to them on both Scales A and B; and the original scales were validated on children aged eight to twelve years, whereas the population in the homes ranged from two to sixteen years. Nonetheless, the prevalence of behaviour problems in the two homes must be regarded as exceptionally high.

Children in the five wards of the paediatric hospital suffered from a variety of diseases and handicaps, of which muscular dystrophy, accounting for 39 per cent, and cerebral palsy, accounting for 21 per cent, were the most common. Although no intelligence test scores were available, it was apparent that many of the children in these wards were of subnormal intelligence, and in 28 per cent of the cases mental subnormality formed part of the diagnosis included in the medical records. For those children who were not deemed subnormal and who were not too ill to attend, schooling was provided by the Local Authority either in the wards themselves or in the two wards converted for school use. Sixty-four per cent of the children received either full-time or part-time education in this way. For the children who were deemed subnormal in the paediatric hospital, there was no educational provision, although some of them might well have benefited.

The children in the subnormality hospital were all severely subnormal. They suffered from a great variety of physical and mental handicaps, the commonest clinical condition being Down's syndrome, or mongolism, which affected 23 per cent. In addition, 12·3 per cent were reported by ward sisters as having marked difficulty with their sight, 4·3 per cent as having marked difficulty with hearing, and 23 per cent were receiving regular treatment by drugs for epilepsy. Mentally, the children were exceedingly backward: 40·7 per cent were profoundly subnormal (IQ 0–20), 52·4 per cent were severely subnormal (IQ 21–50), and only 2·9 per cent were mildly subnormal (IQ more than 50). In 3·9 per cent of the cases, the IQ was unknown.* No child in the subnormality

* No IQ testing was undertaken in the hospital by the research workers, and information on IQ was taken from two sources: the patients' medical records and the records kept by the Psychology Department. Although a programme of routine testing was in operation, many of the test results in medical records were out of date and a variety of tests had been used, yielding different types of scores. Fortunately, at the time of our research, the setting up of an experimental unit required the matching of selected children with controls on IQ, and the Psychology Department had undertaken a review of the records and retested many patients. Even so, several different tests were used, and for many patients a range of IQ scores, or an estimated IQ score was given. Where ranges were specified, we have taken the mean IQ; in the absence of other criteria we have accepted the estimated IQ as though a test had been completed.

hospital was formally educable. Indeed, only 32 per cent attended the hospital training school for severely subnormal children (which was the responsibility of the Health Authority) on a full-time basis. A further 15 per cent attended the school on a half-time or temporary basis, while the remaining children were deemed unsuitable for training, and spent their whole time in the wards.

The procedures for allocating patients to wards in the subnormality hospital resulted in a heavy concentration of the most severely handicapped children in six of the sixteen wards. These six wards, which housed 39 per cent of the total patients, accounted for 65 per cent of the profoundly retarded children (IQ 0–20) and 69 per cent of the children who were unable to walk with or without assistance.* Management problems in these 'low grade' wards were further complicated in that they accounted for 52 per cent of the severely incontinent, 61 per cent of those who had to be fed, 52 per cent of those who had to be dressed, 50 per cent of those who had to be washed, 47 per cent of those with no intelligible speech, and 56 per cent of those who received no schooling at all. It is useful, therefore, to examine these wards separately when comparisons are made with the paediatric hospital.

In the subnormality hospital 55 per cent of the children were able to walk alone and unaided, while 17 per cent were able to walk with the help of others or could get around by crawling or shuffling along the floor. Only 13 per cent of the children in the paediatric wards could walk without assistance, and another 34 per cent were able to move with the help of the staff or with wheelchairs. It can be seen from Table 5.5, however, that the five paediatric wards were closely comparable to the six low-grade subnormality wards in terms of the mobility of the patients.

In several respects, the children in the paediatric wards had abilities which came midway between those of the children in the low-grade and high-grade subnormality wards respectively.

Only about two-fifths of the children in each hospital could feed themselves without assistance and, whether because of inability or lack of opportunity, only 4·2 per cent in the subnormality hospital, and 19·4 per cent in the paediatric hospital, were able to manipulate knives and forks. The details are given in Table 5·6.

Children in the high-grade wards were rather better at dressing themselves than were the children in the paediatric wards, who were in turn more accomplished in this respect than the children in the low-grade wards of the subnormality hospital. Table 5.7

* In an earlier publication, King and Raynes (1968a), p. 42, the proportion of idiot children was wrongly quoted as 57 per cent. Apart from that error, the statistics quoted here for the hospitals differ slightly from those in the earlier report. This is because of a different base date used for the calculations.

TABLE 5.5  *Percentage of children with different degrees of mobility: S.S.N. hospital and paediatric hospital*

| | No. of children | Ambulant[a] | Otherwise mobile[b] | Non-ambulant[c] |
|---|---|---|---|---|
| All wards S.S.N. | 307 | 55·0 | 17·3 | 27·7 |
| 10 high-grade wards S.S.N. | 188 | 74·5 | 11·7 | 13·8 |
| 6 low-grade wards S.S.N. | 119 | 24·3 | 26·4 | 49·3 |
| 5 wards paediatric | 83 | 13·3 | 33·8[d] | 53·1 |

[a]*Ambulant* includes only children able to walk alone and without help.
[b]*Otherwise mobile* includes children who can walk with the help of other people or mechanical aids, and those who are able to move around by means of shuffling, crawling, etc.
[c]*Non-ambulant* includes children who are either bedfast or who are cot and chair patients.
[d]Includes sixteen children who are mobile once they have been helped into wheelchairs.

TABLE 5.6  *Percentages of children with different degrees of ability in feeding: S.S.N. hospital and paediatric hospital*

| | No. children | Use knife and fork | Otherwise feed self | Require help | Have to be fed |
|---|---|---|---|---|---|
| All wards S.S.N. | 307 | 4·2 | 38·8 | 15·3 | 41·7 |
| 10 high-grade wards S.S.N. | 188 | 7·0 | 54·2 | 12·2 | 26·6 |
| 6 low-grade wards S.S.N. | 119 | 0·0 | 14·3 | 20·2 | 65·5 |
| 5 wards paediatric | 83 | 19·4 | 29·8 | 26·3 | 24·6 |

gives the proportions of children with different degrees of ability in this respect.

Much the same picture was found in relation to the abilities of children to wash themselves, as shown in Table 5.8. In both hospitals, feeding, dressing and washing children constituted major problems of management which were largely absent in the two children's homes.

TABLE 5.7  *Percentages of children with different degrees of ability in dressing: S.S.N. hospital and paediatric hospital*

|  | No. children | Able to dress self[a] | Require help | Have to be dressed |
|---|---|---|---|---|
| All wards S.S.N. | 307 | 12·1 | 25·1 | 62·8 |
| 10 high-grade wards S.S.N. | 188 | 18·6 | 31·4 | 50·0 |
| 6 low-grade wards S.S.N. | 119 | 1·7 | 15·1 | 83·3 |
| 5 wards paediatric | 83 | 6·0 | 21·7 | 72·3 |

[a]*Able to dress self* includes children who could dress themselves apart from tying shoe laces and doing up buttons.

TABLE 5.8  *Percentages of children with different degrees of ability in washing: S.S.N. hospital and paediatric hospital*

|  | No. children | Able to wash self | Require help | Have to be washed |
|---|---|---|---|---|
| All wards S.S.N. | 307 | 7·2 | 19·2 | 73·6 |
| 10 high-grade wards S.S.N. | 188 | 11·7 | 28·1 | 60·3 |
| 6 low-grade wards S.S.N. | 119 | 0·0 | 5·0 | 95·0 |
| 5 wards paediatric | 83 | 12·0 | 10·8 | 77·2 |

In respect of two further problems—speech and incontinence—the children in the paediatric hospital were either rather better than those in the subnormality hospital, or else more closely resembled children in the high-grade wards than children in the low-grade wards. Backwardness in speech was a major difficulty in the subnormality hospital. No fewer than 76 per cent of the children had no intelligible speech, while less than 13 per cent could talk even in simple sentences. In the low-grade wards, hardly any children could communicate, except by the use of isolated words. Although the majority of children in the paediatric wards had normal speech, a surprisingly high proportion were retarded in their development. Just over 20 per cent had no intelligible speech, while a further 7 per cent spoke only isolated words, and 8 per cent could use only simple sentences. In this respect, as with incontinence, the children were markedly more handicapped than the children in the homes. These data are presented in Table 5.9.

TABLE 5.9 *Percentages of children with different degrees of ability in speech: S.S.N. hospital and paediatric hospital*

|  | No. children | Normal speech[a] | Simple sentences | Isolated words only | No intelligible speech |
|---|---|---|---|---|---|
| All wards S.S.N. | 309 | 0·0 | 12·4 | 11·4 | 76·2 |
| 10 high-grade wards S.S.N. | 188 | 0·0 | 19·6 | 14·4 | 66·0 |
| 6 low-grade wards S.S.N. | 119 | 0·0 | 0·8 | 6·7 | 92·5 |
| 5 wards paediatric | 83 | 63·9 | 8·4 | 7·2 | 20·5 |

a*Normal speech* includes children who have speech impediments such as stammering, but who are able to conduct conversations without undue difficulty.

No ward in either hospital was free from the problem of incontinence. Less than 16 per cent of the children were clean and dry, and 73 per cent were defined as severely incontinent. In the low-grade wards, no child was fully clean and dry and virtually all of the patients were severely incontinent. Less than two-fifths of the children in the paediatric wards were clean and dry, and about the same proportion were described as severely incontinent.

No systematic study was made of the behavioural problems presented by the children in the two hospitals. It was evident, however, that the subnormality hospital contained very substantial numbers of children who were difficult to manage. While the children in the paediatric hospital were not entirely free of such behavioural problems, antisocial disorders appeared to be uncommon.

To summarize, the four institutions were broadly similar in many respects. The establishments were alike in terms of overall size and the size of the living units, and none of them could be described as overcrowded. By traditional institutional standards the physical facilities were good in all establishments, although the greater number of easy chairs, carpets and private storage facilities in the homes, and the uniformity of decorations and furniture arrangements in the hospitals, gave the former a homely, lived-in appear-

TABLE 5.10 *Percentages of children with different degrees of incontinence: S.S.N. hospital and paediatric hospital*

|  | *No. children* | *Clean and dry* | *Mild incontinence*[a] | *Severe incontinence*[b] |
|---|---|---|---|---|
| All wards S.S.N. | 307 | 15·9 | 11·1 | 73·0 |
| 10 high-grade wards S.S.N. | 188 | 26·1 | 16·5 | 57·4 |
| 6 low-grade wards S.S.N. | 119 | 0·0 | 2·5 | 97·5 |
| 5 wards paediatric | 83 | 39·8 | 22·9 | 37·3 |

[a]*Mild incontinence* is defined as wet nights only or occasional lapses during the day.
[b]*Severe incontinence* is defined as soiled day or night or regularly wet during the day.

ance, while the latter appeared institutional. This impression was reinforced by the sleeping arrangements—small bedrooms for children in the homes, dormitories for the children in the hospitals. The homes were better provided with baths and wash basins, but less well provided with toilets than the hospitals. Again, the institutions were similar in the sex age composition and the length of stay of their residents. In each establishment, there were one or two units for a single sex—usually boys—but for the most part the units had children of both sexes, and with a fairly wide age range. Large differences existed between them in terms of the mental and physical handicaps of the children, with the hospitals sharply marked off from the homes. In many respects, certain units in the subnormality hospital could be directly compared with the units in the paediatric hospital.

# 6 Administration, staffing and patterns of responsibility

The two hospitals were significantly more complex in organizational structure than either of the two children's homes. The hospitals employed larger staffs, who worked in more specialized departments, each with a greater number of hierarchical levels, and linked by less direct and more formalized channels of communication and decision-making. In the non-technical sense of the word, at least, they were more bureaucratic. This may best be shown by consideration of the organization of staffing in the four establishments.

Since the hospitals shared all staff except medical and nursing personnel, it is necessary to consider them together. On 31 January 1964, soon after our fieldwork began, the hospitals employed 892 full-time and 196 part-time staff. These were distributed among five main groupings: administrative and clerical; professional and technical; ancillary; medical; and nursing. Table 6.1 gives the numbers of full-time and part-time staff in each category, together with their equivalent in full-time staff and the permitted 'establishment'.

The hospitals were somewhat understaffed, particularly as far as nurses were concerned, who were seventy below the permitted establishment figure. None the less, the hospitals remained important employers of local labour. A total staff equivalent to 1,008 full-time personnel to care for 675 patients yields an overall ratio of 1·49 staff to every patient. The employment of 551 full-time personnel in administrative, technical and supportive roles, in addition to the 457 doctors and nurses—a ratio of 1·2 other staff to every doctor and nurse—is indicative not only of the size, but also of the complexity of the organizational structure of the hospitals. This complexity can be shown further by an examination of the

TABLE 6.1   *Staff numbers in the two hospitals as at 31 January 1964*

|  | Full-time | Part-time | F-t equiv.* | Establishment |
|---|---|---|---|---|
| Administrative and clerical | 53 | 26 | 67 | 69 |
| Professional and technical | 61 | 9 | 64 | 80 |
| Ancillary | 366 | 78 | 420 | 435 |
| Medical | 23 | 16 | 30 | 31 |
| Nursing | 389 | 67 | 427 | 497 |
| All grades | 892 | 196 | 1,008 | 1,112 |

ªFull-time equivalents are calculated on the basis of a 42-hour week to the nearest whole number.

numbers of specialist departments within the hospitals.

The general administration of the two hospitals was in the hands of the group secretary, who, as well as being the chief executive officer for the group, was also the hospital secretary of both hospitals. There were three central administrative departments, each with a full-time officer in charge. The functions of two of these, finance and supplies, are self-evident. The finance officer was directly responsible to the Hospital Management Committee, while the supplies officer was also the deputy group secretary. The third department, that of the hospital secretary himself, served to co-ordinate the work of all remaining departments in the two hospitals. Each of these central departments employed a number of subordinate administrative and clerical staff, and some of these grades were also found in the professional and ancillary departments in the hospitals.

Sixty-one full-time professional staff were divided between eight major departments: pathology; X-ray; pharmacy; psychology; physiotherapy; speech-therapy; medical social work and medical records. Nine part-time professionals were employed in the following specialisms, although none of them warranted departmental status with an established staff: medical photography; electroencephalography; chiropody; audiometry; and ophthalmology. Ancillary departments employed the equivalent of 420 full-time staff, ranging from the domestic department, with 165 staff—which was the largest—through catering, porters, building, engineering, transport, stores, needle room, central sterile supplies, gardeners, to telephone and reception, which were the smallest.

All of these departments served both the paediatric and the subnormality hospitals: one further department, the training school for the retarded, which employed mainly professional staff, served only the needs of the subnormality hospital.

The head of each department was expected to liaise closely with medical and nursing staff on the wards. Each department employed one or more subordinate grades of staff and, except in those cases where a direct medical responsibility was involved, the head of department was responsible for their work in the first instance to the group secretary, and through him to the Hospital Management Committee.

Although the medical administrator and the matron were appointed to co-ordinate medical and nursing matters for both hospitals, the medical and nursing staffs below this level were quite separate for the two hospitals. Every patient in both hospitals was under the care of a consultant who had the ultimate responsibility for his treatment. In the paediatric hospital there were ten part-time consultants, in addition to the medical administrator, himself a paediatrician. A further six registrars and seven senior house officers completed the ward teams in the various paediatric specialities. Two full-time and three part-time consultants, together with two registrars, were engaged in clinical departments, such as pathology, X-ray and anaesthetics. There was also one part-time dental officer. In the subnormality hospital there were one full-time and two part-time consultants, aided by one senior hospital medical officer,* two senior registrars and two registrars, all of whom were trained in psychological medicine or were undergoing post-graduate training. They treated subnormal patients for minor ailments and injuries, but the usual practice for more serious illnesses was to transfer the patients to a ward in the paediatric hospital.

Nursing staff in the two hospitals were under the control of a single matron, who was assisted in her administrative duties by four assistant matrons, one night superintendent and one night administrative sister.† Of this administrative group, five, including the matron, had been trained in the nursing of sick children, while two had been trained in the nursing of the mentally subnormal. Each of these senior administrative staff took turns in the periodic supervision and inspection of wards in both hospitals, but for the arrangement of the study periods, nurse allocation, staff holidays and off-duty, the administrative nurses specialized in those matters relating to only one hospital or the other.

The nurse training school employed a number of tutors to provide training for the two nursing registers—the Nursing of

* Since 1964 this post has been regraded as 'consultant'.
† At the time of our research, the post of deputy matron was unfilled.

Sick Children (R.S.C.N.) and the Nursing of the Mentally Subnormal (R.N.M.S.). A further administrative sister was employed
to take charge of the nurses' home, where the resident staff lived.
All other nurses were to be found on the wards of the two hospitals,
or in specialized departments, including the operating theatre.

TABLE 6.2    *Mean weekly numbers of ward nursing staff in two*
*hospitals: January to March 1964*[a]

| Grade of staff | Paediatric | | S.S.N. | |
|---|---|---|---|---|
| | No. | % | No. | % |
| Ward sisters and charge nurses | 38 | 14·2 | 30 | 20·6 |
| Staff nurses | 26 | 9·8 | 10 | 6·8 |
| Students[b] | 165 | 62·0 | 41 | 28·1 |
| Assistants and auxiliaries[c] | 37 | 14·0 | 65 | 44·5 |
| All grades | 266 | 100·0 | 146 | 100·0 |

[a]Figures are given in full-time equivalents.
[b]Includes eight students in the paediatric hospital and four in the subnormality
hospital who were undergoing post-graduate training, having already qualified
for another nursing register.
[c]Includes three State enrolled nurses in the paediatric hospital who had undergone
a two-year training.

Table 6.2, which lists the average numbers of staff in the two
hospitals for the period January to March 1964, gives some indication of the number of different status levels within the nursing
hierarchy, although these have been simplified slightly for ease of
presentation.

A fuller account of the organization of the two hospitals and
the patterns of responsibility within them is given by King (1970).
However, it should be apparent from the foregoing that what
happened in the wards was the result of the complex co-ordination
of the activities of three separate hierarchies: the administrative,
the medical and the nursing. In brief, ward sisters and charge
nurses were responsible to the matron for the day-to-day management of their wards, and to the consultants and doctors for the
carrying-out of the prescribed treatments. Junior nursing staff were
responsible to the matron, through the ward sisters and the charge
nurses. Departmental heads were expected to liaise closely with the
nursing and medical staff of the wards, but were responsible to
the hospital secretary for the work in their departments. Final
responsibility for the health and welfare of the patients was vested
in the consultant medical staff, who admitted them.

The two children's homes, by contrast, were very much simpler in their organizational structure, and employed many fewer staff. Table 6.3 shows the close similarity between the staffing of the two institutions, and for some purposes they can be conveniently described together. Between them, they employed the equivalent of 255 full-time staff to care for 717 children—an overall ratio of 0·36 staff to every child, compared to a ratio of 1·49 staff to every patient in the hospitals. Unlike the hospitals, they employed fewer staff in administrative, technical and other supportive roles than in direct child-care duties; there were the equivalent of 110 full-time personnel in the former category and 145 in the latter— a ratio of 0·76 other staff to every member of the child-care staff, compared to a ratio of 1·2 other staff to one medical or nursing staff in the hospitals.

TABLE 6.3   *Staff numbers in two homes*

|  | First home (1-1-64) | | | Second home (1-3-64) | | |
|  | Full-time | Part-time | F-t. equiv[a] | Full-time | Part-time | F-t. equiv.[a] |
|---|---|---|---|---|---|---|
| Administrative and clerical | 9 | — | 9 | 9 | — | 9 |
| Professional and technical | 9 | — | 9 | 11 | 1 | 12 |
| Ancillary | 7 | 41 | 31 | 12 | 56 | 40 |
| Child-care | 70 | — | 70 | 75 | — | 75 |
| All grades | 95 | 41 | 119 | 107 | 57 | 136 |

[a]Full-time equivalents are calculated on the basis of a 42-hour week to the nearest whole number.

The homes were each administered by a superintendent, appointed by the Children's Department of the Local Authority, who was both chief executive for the organization and head of the child-care staff. He was assisted by a deputy superintendent and a matron and deputy matron, who completed the administrative staff. There was no separate lay administrative hierarchy as there was in the hospitals: a good deal of responsibility for routine administration was devolved upon cottage staff, more general matters being dealt with by the superintendent or matron. Child-care staff in the establishments were responsible to their respective superintendent, or, where powers had been appropriately delegated, to the matron.

There was comparatively little specialization of function among the ancillary grades of staff, and little in the way of departmental

F

organization. Domestics—the largest group of ancillary staff, for example—were mostly part-time, non-resident workers under the supervision of the matron, and without a separate departmental head. In addition to the domestic staff, there were a number of storekeepers, drivers, seamstresses, shoemakers and repairers, gardeners and engineers employed in each establishment. These were not formalized into departments, however, and the usual pattern was for one or two full-time, higher-grade employees to supervise a number of part-time employees. Ancillary staff were directly responsible for their activities to either the superintendent or the matron.

A small group of trained nurses was attached to the sick-bay in each establishment. For general medical, dental and other services, the homes used the normal community services in their area, and had special arrangements with nearby hospitals for specialist psychiatric and optical services.

### Staffing and responsibility in the living units

Since our main concern is with the daily care of children, more detailed attention needs to be given to the structure and organization of the living units in which they spent most of their time.

### *Staffing*

The wards in both hospitals were staffed by nurses. There were some differences in numbers, training and organization of staff between the two hospitals. It can be seen from Table 6.2 that there were, on average, 266 nurses of all grades actually assigned to wards in the paediatric hospital for the period January to March 1964. In those months the bed occupancy for the hospital averaged 395 patients, so that what we have called the *assigned* staff to child ratio was 1:1·48. In the subnormality hospital during the same period, the figures were 146 nurses of all grades to 307 patients, giving an *assigned* staff to children ratio of 1:2·1. Not only did the paediatric hospital have more nurses than the subnormality hospital, but a higher proportion of them had also completed, or were undergoing, training: 87·4 per cent of the nurses in the paediatric hospital were in this category, or one for every 1·7 children, as against 55·5 per cent for those in the subnormality hospital, or one for every 3·8 children. These crude ratios of assigned staff, however, give little real indication of the staffing in the wards, since they take no account of holidays, sickness, off-duty and the rotation of student nurses from ward to ward in the course of their training.

In both hospitals, sisters and charge nurses were permanently allocated to their own wards, and many had worked on the same ward for several years. Staff nurses were also allocated to their own wards, at least in theory, but they were frequently required to change wards whenever the absence of a sister or a charge nurse—through sickness or holidays—left only junior staff on a ward. Student nurses were expected to spend three months on each of a number of wards in order to meet the requirements laid down by the General Nursing Council for their training, and also to spend three months on night duty. Other staff—State enrolled nurses, nursing auxilliaries or assistants—were not permanently allocated to particular wards, but were used to fill in the gaps where they were most needed.

Allocation to the wards for students and untrained nurses was arranged by the Administrative Nursing Office, and was communicated to staff by means of a list, known as the 'change list', which was posted in the nurses' home. This list, drawn up by the assistant matrons in collaboration with the nursing tutors, informed nurses of the wards on which they would be expected to work the following week, as well as any study periods allocated to them. Students in the paediatric hospital spent an initial period of eight weeks in the nurse training school, followed by training in the wards, interspersed with several 'study blocks' of three or four weeks each in the course of the three years. Students in the subnormality hospital also spent an initial eight-week period in the school, but thereafter spent one study day a week at school, and received the rest of their training in the wards. Students in fact spent rather less than the intended three months on each ward required for their training: in the subnormality hospital the average time spent on each ward was 8·2 weeks, while the average for students in the paediatric hospital was 10·2 weeks. Some untrained staff spent several years on the same ward, while others were subject to ward changes every few weeks. In general, they spent rather longer on the wards than did students in training, but in both hospitals there was considerable turnover in staffing as between wards.

Nursing staff were organized in different ways in the paediatric and subnormality hospitals. Throughout the subnormality hospital, two equal senior members of staff were allocated to each ward. Some wards had two sisters, others two charge nurses, and still others one sister and one charge nurse. These two senior staff shared responsibility for their ward, although they were always on duty at different times. Each week, the sister or charge nurse on duty examined the change list, to see who was allocated to the ward the following week, and then submitted arrangements for staff off-duty periods to the administrative office. Two alternative systems of duty arrangements were available, both based on a fortnightly cycle. In the first, staff worked on a shift basis; under this system, staff worked five mornings (from 7.30 a.m. until 2 p.m.), with one long day (7.30 a.m. until 6 p.m.) and one day off in the first week, and five afternoons (from 12.30 p.m. until 8.30 p.m.) with one long day and one day off in the second week. The alternative involved staff working on a long-day basis: under this system, staff worked four long days (from 7.30 a.m. until 8.30 p.m.) with three days off in the first week, and three long days with four days off in the second. Both systems produced an average working week of forty-two hours, and the choice of systems was left to the ward staff. In practice, all but two wards worked to the shift system. At night the wards were staffed by one night nurse from 8.15 p.m. until 7.30 a.m. Although an attempt was made to keep the same night nurse for the same ward, there were as many ward changes for night staff as there were for day staff.

In addition to the senior staff, each subnormality ward would normally be allocated four or five nurses, of whom three or four would be untrained nursing assistants, and one or two trained staff nurses or students in training. Exceptionally, wards with children who were seen as easy to manage might be allocated only three nurses, while difficult wards might be allocated six nurses. In January 1964 the mean weekly allocation of nurses to subnormality wards was 4·75. Not all of these, however, would be on duty at the same time and due allowance has to be made both for off-duty periods and study days. When allowance is made for these factors, both the shift system and the long-day system produced similar staff availability during the morning and afternoon periods, with, usually, three members of staff, including the sister or charge nurse, on duty. Exceptionally, this might be as low as two or as high as four. However, the shift system, which was in fact the most popular, did not cover the evening period as well as the long-day system, because each day one member of staff left the ward at 6 p.m. This meant that two staff were left on duty between 6 p.m. and 8.30 p.m. on the shift system, as opposed to three members of staff under the long-day system.

When staff allocation, off-duty arrangements and study days are taken into account, what we have called *effective* staff–child ratios can be calculated—that is, the ratio of staff on duty at particular times to the numbers of patients at those times. On this basis, mean *effective* staff–child ratios for the wards in the subnormality hospital in January 1964 were as follows: 1 : 6·4 during the mornings, 1 : 6·53 in the afternoons, 1 : 10·81 in the early evenings and 1 : 19·2 at night. On the wards where some of the children went to the training school, these ratios would be improved for two hours in the morning and two hours in the afternoon. The subnormality hospital was thus somewhat better staffed than those reported by Morris (1969).*

In the paediatric hospital, only one ward sister was allocated to each ward on a permanent basis. The sister was responsible for her ward to the matron, and, at times when she was not on duty, the ward was handed over to a trained staff nurse or to a third-year student. Each ward was again allocated junior staff through the medium of the change list on a weekly basis. The numbers of staff allocated to the wards each week depended on the type of ward; shortstay, acute surgical and medical wards received more staff than the longstay medical wards. In January 1964 shortstay wards received, on average, 10·33 nurses in addition to the sister; longstay wards received 4·25 nurses in addition to the sister. Of the ten or so staff allocated weekly to the shortstay wards, at least one would be a trained staff nurse, and the remainder would usually be student nurses in training. Occasionally, one or two untrained nurses would be included in the team. For the longstay wards, the staffing pattern was similar to the subnormality hospital: of the four or five staff allocated, one or two would be trained nurses or students, while three or four would be untrained.

All of the wards in the paediatric hospital worked a 'split-duty' system, under which staff worked from 7.30 a.m. until 8.30 p.m. for five days each week, with a break of two hours in the morning and two hours in the afternoon. This system was complicated by the fact that some untrained nurses were allowed to work a long-day system if they preferred, and a few individuals were

* The ratio of assigned ward nurses to patients in this study was 1:2·1, whereas the mean for thirty-four hospitals studied by Morris (1969) was 1:4·7 and the best ratio she found was 1:2·9. Her figures are not strictly comparable to ours, since she includes administrative nurses who do not work on wards, and thus the ratios she quotes appear marginally better than they really are. On the other hand, her figures relate to hospitals caring for adults as well as children, and adult wards are typically worse off for staff than wards for children. Morris does not quote assigned ratios for children's wards, but gives instead ratios which are based on the numbers of staff on duty at the time of the visit by her research team (always between 9 a.m. and 6 p.m.). These figures are thus nearly comparable to our effective staff ratios, which for the morning period were 1:6·4 and for the afternoon 1:6·53. Unfortunately, the weighted average quoted by Morris is misleading – it appears to be weighted for the size of hospitals, thus including adult units, rather than for the size of the children's wards – and it is not possible, therefore, to quote an average statistic for the data she gives. However, of the thirty-one hospitals having children's units which she visited, twenty-two had worse staff ratios at the time of her visit, and nine had better staff ratios than the hospital discussed here. The range she found was from 1:5 to 1:19·4. See Morris (1969), pp. 105, 106, Table 6.2.

allowed to work on a shift system, similar to that operating in the subnormality wards. At night, the longstay wards in the paediatric hospital were staffed by one night nurse, while the shortstay wards were staffed by two night nurses.

Because of the complicated way in which off-duty time was taken under the split-duty system, it is not possible to break down the day into convenient periods for the assessment of *effective* staffing ratios in the way this was done for the subnormality hospital. Usually, staff took their off-duty periods in rotation, so that only one member of the team on duty for the day would be away from the ward at any one time. This meant that for most of the day shortstay wards had five or six nurses on duty, while longstay wards had three nurses on duty, including the ward sister. When staff ratios are calculated on the basis of approximate numbers of staff actually on duty, therefore, this system resulted in one member of staff for 3·2 children for most of the day on the shortstay wards and one member of staff for 5·34 children on the longstay wards. Both ratios compare favourably with the best staff ratios in the subnormality hospital. The split-duty system provided more adequate coverage of the wards than either the shift system or the long-day system, although many of the staff in the paediatric hospital complained that the periods of two hours off-duty in the middle of the day were really wasted, since they had no time to leave the hospital.

The method of staffing the cottages of the two children's homes was very different from the hospitals. Table 6.4 gives the numbers for each grade of staff working in cottages during our initial field-work periods at the two establishments.

TABLE 6.4  *Numbers of cottage child-care staff in two homes*

| Grade of staff | First home | | Second home | |
|---|---|---|---|---|
| | No. | % | No. | % |
| Housemothers | 22 | 31·4 | 36 | 48·0 |
| Housefathers | 5 | 7·1 | 1 | 1·3 |
| Deputy housemothers | 17 | 24·3 | 0 | 0·0 |
| Assistant housemothers | 23 | 32·9 | 36 | 48·0 |
| Students | 3 | 4·3 | 2 | 2·7 |
| All grades | 70 | 100·0 | 75 | 100·0 |

In both homes, each cottage was in the charge of a housemother permanently assigned to that unit. Thirty-two per cent of housemothers at the first home, and 17 per cent at the second, were married women whose husbands lived with them in the units. Occasionally, the husbands were employed by the institutions as housefathers, and in such cases the married couple shared the responsibility for their household. There were five such living units in the first home and one in the second. More usually, the husband pursued a full-time occupation elsewhere, and would help out in the cottage during the evenings, even though not a full-time member of staff. More than 80 per cent of the housemothers in both establishments had worked in the same unit for a year or longer and many of them had had five or more years of experience in the same cottage, where they had watched the children grow up.

In the first home, there were two additional grades of child-care staff attached to cottages—deputy housemothers and assistant housemothers. The post of deputy housemother was a new grading, introduced by this institution in an attempt to make the career prospects for this kind of work more attractive. Deputies carried somewhat more responsibility and had a slightly higher salary than assistants. The grade of deputy housemother did not exist in the second home, where all junior staff were referred to as assistant housemothers. At the time in question, there were no male junior staff in either home, although there had been some deputy housefathers in the first home prior to our study, and a few assistant housefathers have been appointed since.

Junior staff were also allocated permanently to cottages, and the policy of both establishments was to keep the staff in the same unit, unless severe problems of relationship between staff and children arose. Even so, 56 per cent of the deputies and 84 per cent of the assistants in the first home had worked in the same unit for less than a year. In the second home, 55 per cent of the junior staff had worked in the same unit for a similar period. In both cases, these figures reflect the high turnover of junior staff in the two homes, rather than transfers between units, since less than a quarter of the junior staff in each home had worked on two or more units during their stay. Although there were some changes during the course of our investigation, for the most part the staffing position in the cottages was as follows: in the first home, four cottages had three members of staff in addition to the housemother; three cottages had only one assistant; while the remaining fifteen cottages had two additional members of staff. In the second home, all except two of the units had only one assistant in addition to the housemother; one unit was run by a married couple with no further help; and one unit, which had a higher proportion of younger children, had two assistant staff.

The smaller numbers of staff in the cottages in the second

home were matched, of course, by the smaller numbers of children in each cottage, so that there was little difference between the crude ratios of *assigned* cottage staff to children for the two homes. The mean *assigned* ratio for the first home was 1:5·08 children, while that for the second home was 1:5·14 children. The crude ratios of cottage-based staff to children compare very unfavourably with those quoted earlier for ward-based staff to patients in the two hospitals. However, these assigned ratios, like those for the hospitals, take no account of the organization of staffing within the units. When factors such as the hours of duty, holidays and sickness are taken into account, the differences between the hospitals and the homes are greatly reduced, largely because the homes did not employ staff on a shift basis, and their staff were required to work much longer hours. Even so, it is clear that staff were considerably stretched to provide tolerably acceptable staff ratios.

One of the major differences between the hospitals and the homes was that virtually all of the full-time child-care staff in the homes were themselves resident in the cottages in which they worked, whereas no hospital staff lived in their units. Officially, all grades of staff were expected to work a five-day week of sixty-five hours, with two days off each week. For the five working days, staff worked a system of duty not unlike the split-duty system at the paediatric hospital, except that longer hours were involved. Staff came on duty at 7 a.m. and remained on duty until 2 p.m., at which point they had a two-hour break. They then worked from 4 p.m. until 10 p.m. Most of the children went to school in the mornings and the afternoons, returning to their cottages for a meal at midday. The units were thus at their busiest during the early morning, at midday and again in the late afternoon and evenings. During the late morning lunches had to be prepared, and the staff break was thus taken during the slackest period in the afternoon. Staff were 'on call' during this break, however, and so were not able to leave the establishment. Staff were also on call at night, thus obviating the need for special night staff.

This system of duties ensured that the maximum number of the available staff were actually on duty in the cottages when the children were present, but even in normal times allowance has to be made for the two days off each week to which each member of staff was entitled. Allowing for days of off-duty, the maximally efficient arrangement of staff produces the following patterns: a cottage with two permanent members of staff would have both of them on duty at the times when children were present in the unit for only three days each week, but have four days when one member had to cope alone. A unit with three staff had two of them on duty for six days and all three on duty for the seventh. A unit with four staff had three members on for six days in the week and two members on for the seventh. On this basis, effective staff ratios for cottages in the first home ranged from 1:15 for four days a week in one cottage at its worst, to 1:4·3 for six days a week in another cottage at its best. The 'typical' cottage, with three members of staff and fifteen children, would have ratios of 1:5 for one day each week and of 1:7·5 for the other six days. In the second home, where the typical cottage had two members of staff and ten children, the effective ratios would be 1:5 for three days each week and 1:10 for four days.

What is striking about the staffing of the units is that neither home had spare staff available to cope with the problems of illness and holidays. Both homes had a few student housemothers not directly attached to the living units, who could be used in emergencies; at the time of our research, there were three students at the first home and two at the second. For the most part, however, holidays and sickness meant that the unit concerned carried on with what staff remained. It is perhaps not surprising that the turnover of staff, particularly among assistants, was high.

Comparatively few of the total staff in either home had received a formal training for their work: 53 per cent of all staff in the first home and 35 per cent in the second were untrained. Most of the housemothers, however, in both homes, had received some kind of training; three-fifths in the first home and three-quarters in the second. Only 23 per cent of housemothers in the first home and 31 per cent in the second had received the full one-year Home Office Training Course, the remainder having received part-time refresher courses or an in-service training. These findings are consistent with those reported by Monsky (1963).

*Responsibility*

The hospitals also differed markedly from the children's homes in the patterns of authority and responsibility which obtained within the living units. This was most noticeable when the roles of what we have called the *head of the unit*—sisters and charge nurses in the hospitals and housemothers in the homes—were compared, and when parts played by junior staff in both types of establishment were analysed. There were a number of subtle differences between the paediatric hospital and the subnormality hospital, as well as between each of the homes, but for simplicity the contrast here will be made between the hospitals on the one hand and the homes on the other.

The staff in each establishment were asked a series of questions about who was responsible for the final decision in a number of matters affecting the staff and children in the living units. In each case, they were required to say who had made the decision on the last occasion it occurred and what degree of consultation had taken place before the decision was taken.

In two respects, there was comparatively little difference between the homes and the hospitals. Firstly, decisions relating to the immediate or future welfare of the children were removed from the area of responsibility of unit heads in both homes and hospitals. The decision to move a child to another unit, or to send a child to school, or for a period of home leave, for example, were taken by the medical or professional staff of the hospitals and by the superintendent or matron in the homes. However, the usual practice in the homes was for these matters to be discussed with unit heads first, often at their instigation, whereas in the hospitals ward staff complained that they might learn of the decision only through the receipt of a memorandum or when someone with authority came to remove the child from the ward. Secondly, decisions relating to staff, once basic allocations to units had been made, were very much in the hands of unit heads in both establishments. Thus either ward sisters or charge nurses and house-mothers could determine the allocation of particular jobs to junior staff, as well as the details of off-duty arrangements. But here, too, there were differences in the way these were carried out. In the homes, the allocation of tasks to junior staff was a matter of discussion and agreement between those involved: in the hospitals, the allocation of duties followed very much the pattern of seniority and status within the nursing hierarchy. In much the same way, off-duty days in the children's homes were decided by discussion and compromise, whereas in the hospitals the more favoured off-duty days tended to go with seniority and status.

In two other respects, the differences between the hospitals and the homes were more striking. Much of the responsibility for deciding the daily routine of the living units which was given to houseparents in the homes was denied to ward sisters by the nature of the wider organization. Meals in the children's homes were cooked by cottage staff in the household kitchen. Meals could thus be taken at the convenience of staff and children in the cottages, earlier on some occasions than on others. In the hospitals, on the other hand, all cooked meals were prepared in central kitchens and delivered to wards by the hospital porters. The timing of meals was thus decided centrally, but wide margins had to be allowed to take account of delivery time. As a result, ward staff had to gear their routine to the expected time of arrival of the meals. In a similar way, the heads of units in the hospitals had less discretion in determining the times at which children got up and went to bed. In theory, these times were defined in standing orders, issued centrally by the matron and applicable to all wards in both hospitals. In practice, they were determined by the duty hours of staff. Children were got up in the mornings before day staff came on duty and were put to bed in the evenings before the night staff arrived. The exact timing depended on the number of staff available to deal with the number of children present, but there was little scope for individual decision. In the homes, where staff were resident and where the distinction between 'off-duty' and 'on-call' was, to say the least, sometimes blurred, unit heads had a good deal of discretion in deciding the bed-times of individual children. In many other respects too, the daily routine of the hospital wards was defined by standing orders.

Much the most important differences, however, between the hospitals and the homes were in the amount of authority delegated to unit heads to purchase goods either for the children or for their units. In the hospitals, such matters as buying clothes or toys for the children were dealt with centrally by the supplies department, and the unit heads simply requisitioned items as and when needed. They had little or no choice in the kinds of items provided. They had no petty cash allowance to make direct purchases themselves. Occasionally, when special monies became available as a result of gifts or bequests, ward sisters might be consulted as to the kind of equipment required in their wards. In the homes, a great deal of responsibility was devolved upon the houseparents. Within certain limits, cash or credit allowances were available to purchase clothes for the children, and to purchase toys. These could be bought either from stores within each establishment, or from local shops at which the homes had accounts. Houseparents were usually able to take the children with them to make the purchases, and for the most part they had a reasonable degree of choice from a range of alternatives. In the homes, this responsibility for making purchases was further extended so that each housemother was given a weekly housekeeping allowance from which she was able to buy food and household goods for the unit. Again, items could either be bought through stores within the establishment or from outside shops. Most housemothers, for example, had regular weekly orders with the local milkman, baker, grocer and greengrocer, who delivered goods to the cottages. No such responsibilities were extended to the heads of units within the hospitals. Food, household goods, cleaning materials and so on were requisitioned by ward sisters or charge nurses on a daily or weekly basis from the relevant central department within the hospital.

These differences in the amount of responsibility and discretion given to unit heads are reflected in the system of central supervision of the living units. Each ward in the hospitals was routinely visited by representatives from the administrative nursing office at least twice, and often three times, during the day, and at least once and often twice during the night. In addition to these routine visits, at which written reports of the state of the ward were presented, wards were periodically inspected by the matron. In the homes, no regular routine visits occurred. The superintendents and matrons, of course, could have access whenever they wished, but in practice came only when there were real matters to discuss.

There were also differences between hospitals and homes in the way in which junior staff were integrated within their units. Some differences have already been mentioned, such as the greater degree of consultation that was reported by staff in the homes, when such matters as off-duty and other arrangements were made. But some differences were even more marked. Clear distinctions could be observed in the hospitals between the type of work done by different grades of ward staff. Some jobs, such as toileting the children, were performed by senior ward staff only when no other staff were available to cope, while others, such as checking laundry deliveries, were reserved for more senior members of the unit. The distinctions of role were symbolized in the many subtle variations in colour and design of uniforms which distinguished each grade of staff. The differences between roles of particular grades of staff transcended ward boundaries, so that there would be greater similarities between the activities of student nurses on two different wards than between the activities of a student nurse and a nursing assistant on the same ward. Moreover, these status distinctions were reinforced outside the wards: separate facilities, sitting rooms and diningrooms were provided for sisters and other staff in the nurses' home, and separate annual dances were held.

In the children's homes there was very little specialization of roles as between staff. Although housemothers took responsibility for buying goods and other administrative duties, they could also be found cooking meals, dusting furniture and washing and caring for the children. In effect, the roles of junior staff tended to vary from cottage to cottage, and to reflect 'the way things are done' in their own particular unit. No uniforms were worn and both senior and junior staff would wear similar nylon overalls. There were few facilities outside the cottages where status distinctions could be enforced; and both housemothers and assistants lived in the cottages where they worked. For both grades of staff, the accommodation was poor and cramped, especially in the first home. Housemothers usually had a bedroom and a sittingroom to themselves; assistants had only a small bed-sittingroom.

# 7 Patterns of care

In each of the living units studied, observations were made by
the two sociologists at different times and on different days so
that a composite picture of life in the units during weekdays, weekends and holidays, and from early morning throughout the day and
during the nights, could be built up. Systematic and repeated
observations were undertaken of meal-times, toilet routines, bathing
and other procedures. After much preliminary and informal discussions and piloting, a pre-coded interview schedule was developed,
designed to elicit information about day-to-day activities in the
units. Wherever possible, questions were asked about specific situations occurring on the day before the interview took place, and it
was frequently possible to check interview responses against independent observations. To enhance reliability, and to ensure greater
comparability between establishments, many questions were restricted to specific children, randomly selected from each unit, and all
of whom were fully ambulant. Most of the questions were factual
and highly detailed; no respondent in any establishment refused to
co-operate, and considerable confidence was felt by the research
workers in the validity of responses.*

Most of the data were collected with the intention of quantifying
differences between the establishments, and an attempt to characterize the institutions in quantitative terms is presented in Chapter 8.
Here we are concerned to describe some of the differences in the
patterns of care. Perhaps these may best be portrayed by considering certain routine aspects of life in each. Once again, the two

* See Appendices II and III. To avoid too much repetition, only the instruments
used in the final survey (described in Part III) are presented in the Appendices. All
of the instruments used in the survey were developed from those used in the field
studies, with only slight modification. Full details of reliability are given there.

homes were so alike, and the two hospitals so similar, that the contrasts may be drawn between homes on the one hand and hospitals on the other. Only occasionally will it be necessary to distinguish between the paediatric and the subnormality hospitals.

## The children's day

The day begins with waking and getting dressed. In eleven units of the subnormality hospital, washing and dressing the children was the responsibility of a night nurse: the children were toileted and dressed and made ready for breakfast before the day staff came on duty. The night nurse therefore had the task of coping with up to twenty handicapped children — and the job had to be finished by 7.30 a.m. Because of frequent changes in night staff (in one typical ward, for example, forty-two different night nurses were on duty in the course of a single year), the nurse would, more often than not, be dealing with children whom she did not know. The usual practice was therefore to go from bed to bed, waking each child in turn and taking him to the toilet or sitting him on a pot in the ward. Since one nurse could not cope with more than a few children at a time, each child was then washed and dressed and returned to his or her bed. All of this, of course, takes time; and in two wards the process started between 4 and 5 a.m., while in another nine it began soon after 5 a.m. In the remaining five wards of this hospital, night staff were not responsible for dressing the children and after waking, toileting and washing them, the night nurse put the children back to bed in their nightdresses. In these wards the process began about 6 a.m.

Night nurses in the paediatric hospital were not usually required to dress the children. In three wards the night nurse began getting the children up at 6 a.m., while in the other two wards the children were not wakened until after 6.30 a.m.

What did those children who had been early in the queue for being dressed, many of whom were extremely active, do until the day staff came on duty? To answer this question, inquiries were made about the random sample of ambulant children in each ward. In about two wards in five, in both hospitals, the children merely remained in or on their beds with nothing to do. In other wards, however, some attempt was made to provide the children with toys or books in the dormitory, but much depended on the initiative of the night nurse on duty. There was only one ward in the subnormality hospital where the children were allowed to leave the dormitory and go into the dayroom before the day staff arrived.

Getting-up times in both hospitals were the same at weekends as during the week — indeed, except for those children who went to school during the week, ward routine remained much the same throughout the year.

In the children's homes, most of the children could dress themselves, and no night staff were employed. With some variation from one cottage to another, the children were wakened between 6.45 and 7.30 a.m. Those children with furthest to go to school or to work were wakened first. The children washed and dressed themselves and came downstairs to breakfast as soon as they were ready. The younger children were helped by the housemother or her assistant. There was little time to waste in the mornings, although many children played with particular toys while they waited for breakfast to arrive. On Saturdays, and in particular on Sundays, however, things were very different. Getting up was anything from a quarter of an hour to two hours later than during the week. The children and the staff would have a 'lie in'.

Breakfast also differed between the establishments. In both hospitals, bread and butter and cereals for breakfast were prepared in the kitchens on each ward, usually by the night staff, while the children were asleep. The cooked part of the meal was prepared in the central kitchen and delivered to the wards in hot containers. This had the disadvantage for the children that they rarely, if ever, saw food being prepared. Although snacks and drinks were prepared on the wards later in the day while children were present, few children were permitted to enter the kitchen to watch. A further disadvantage for the children was that they were required to sit at tables before the breakfast arrived, and since it was often late being delivered they frequently had to wait at tables for up to twenty minutes before they could begin to eat. The ambulant children sat at small tables, with three or four children to each, and plates of food were brought to them by the staff. On no occasion did the staff ever eat with the children, or sit down with them at table. Since staff were not permitted to take their own meals in the wards, except on Christmas Day, the children, while they remained in the hospital, had no opportunity to watch adults eat and to learn from the experience. Non-ambulant children and difficult feeders in both hospitals were fed either in their beds, or in special chairs, by the staff. This pattern was repeated at all meals, which were always taken at the same times throughout the week and at weekends.

In the children's homes, all the cooking and preparation was undertaken in the cottages by the housemothers and assistants. Most cottages required that children organize themselves to help, either in the preparation of meals or, more frequently, in the setting of tables, washing up and other similar tasks. In other cottages, the children could help if they wished. At least one member of staff always ate with the children at all meals and in all cottages. Food was served from the table by the staff. In some cottages, staff had separate crockery and separate plates of bread and butter from the children, but this practice was comparatively rare. In many cottages, breakfast was a rather straggling affair, with some children having finished and left almost before others had started. This pattern, too, held good for other meals during the day, and there was a good deal of variation in meal-times at weekends, particularly in the case of 'Sunday lunch'.

After breakfast, and after every other meal, the children in the subnormality hospital were taken to the toilets. Only one ward in the paediatric hospital, containing mainly older children, did not observe this ritual. Toileting was clearly a major problem in a hospital in which over four-fifths of the children were incontinent, or where, as in the paediatric wards, although two-fifths of the children could recognize their own needs to go to the w.c., more than 90 per cent were dependent upon staff for their toileting because of their physical handicaps. Two subnormal wards and one paediatric ward toileted children only after meals—three times a day—as a matter of routine. The great majority of wards in both hospitals, however, required that all children went to the toilet at more frequent intervals, regardless of need, so that a most noticeable feature of ward routine was the amount of time spent by children in the toilets—for some children about three hours daily. Seven subnormality wards and one paediatric ward toileted the children as often as six times during the day, two subnormal and one paediatric ward toileted them five times, and five subnormal and one paediatric ward toileted them four times.

In the wards where toileting was more frequent, not every child was required to attend all toilet sessions, some of which were restricted to the severely incontinent only. In all wards, however, some children were toileted as necessary in addition to the routine sessions. There was a slight tendency for the wards with the most severely incontinent children to have more frequent toilet sessions than those with less severely incontinent children, but the tendency was not marked. No such tendency could be observed in the paediatric wards, although the one ward which had no set routine sessions was, in fact, the one with the fewest incontinent children.

For the toilet sessions which followed main meals, the usual practice in wards where most of the children were ambulant was for children to wait at the tables until all had finished eating and the plates had been cleared away. This, for some children, could mean a difficult period of waiting for about a quarter of an hour or twenty minutes. Some overactive children had to be loosely tied to their chairs to restrain them during this time. Then, all the ambulant children were led out to the toilets together. While the children were in the toilet annexe, one member of staff would sweep and tidy the dayroom. For other toilet sessions there was some variation from ward to ward in the method of organization. In seven subnormality wards, all of the ambulant children were always taken to the toilet together; there they remained until the toilet routine had been completed, when they were all returned to the dayroom as one large group. In the other nine wards, the treatment was somewhat more individual, with children being either taken to, or returned from, the toilets in smaller groups, though even in these wards there was usually a heavy concentration of ambulant children in the toilets at the same time. Non-ambulant children, of necessity, received still more individual treatment. They were usually carried to the toilets and returned immediately they had finished or else they were potted or changed in the dormitory. In the paediatric wards, where most of the children were non-ambulant, the more active children were taken to the toilets a group at a time.

While the children were in the toilets, they were supervised by two or three members of staff, although this might often be reduced to only one nurse. Some children would sit on w.c.s, other on chamber pots. Many would run around naked or sit on the floor. It was often difficult to tell which child was supposed to be where, and occasionally the same child could be observed being toileted twice by different members of staff. If more than one member of staff was on duty in the toilets, it was usual for them to divide their activities so that what we have called the *conveyor-belt system* was operated: one nurse would toilet a child and hand him over to another nurse for washing and drying. Just over half the wards in each hospital regularly used the conveyor-belt system, and several other wards used it on some occasions.

In one mental subnormality ward, a sister claimed the children were never left on a lavatory or chamber pot for longer than ten minutes; but another sister said she left them there 'for an hour or more if necessary'. In some wards the toilet session would be as short as twenty minutes, while on others sessions lasted an hour or more. However, even on a ward which had relatively few toilet sessions, a child could expect to spend up to an hour and a half a day in the toilet, while on a ward which had many sessions a child might spend two or three hours a day in the toilets. In wards where feeding as well as toileting was a problem, meals and toileting might leave little time for anything else.

In the children's homes, of course, the problems of toileting during the day scarcely arose. A few of the youngest children required some assistance or oversight in respect of toilet needs, but the older children were well able to look after themselves. Children used the toilets whenever they needed to, and not as the result of a routinely organized session. In any case, the toilets were separate and enclosed, which afforded a degree of privacy which was never found in the hospitals.

After breakfasting and toileting in the subnormality hospital, the schoolchildren were got ready for school. In the six low-grade wards only about one-fifth of the children went to the training school, mostly for the morning session only; in the ten high-grade wards, about three-fifths of the children went to school, mostly for both mornings and afternoons. The remaining children stayed behind on the wards. The schoolchildren were the only ones provided with hospital topcoats, since they were the only ones to have cause to be outside in bad weather. The ward staff dressed them in 'outside' clothes and the children waited in the corridor until it was time to go to school. They were then taken by a nurse, or occasionally collected by a teacher, and led crocodile fashion along the central avenue to the school. They returned two hours later in the same way. At the school, a great deal of activity took place: but the classes were overcrowded (14·6 as against the recommended 10 per class), and the buildings were old and inadequate.

For those who stayed behind on the wards, there was little to do. If it was fine, they were allowed to play in the courtyard, under the supervision of the staff. If it was wet or cold, they remained in the dayroom. A drink of orange squash or milk was provided at midmorning for the non-school children. Those children who were not active could often be observed for long periods with no social contacts at all. Much the same pattern was repeated during school hours in the afternoon.

In the paediatric wards, almost all of the children, except those who also suffered from some degree of subnormality, received some form of education. Most of the children were taught in their wards by visiting teachers from the Local Education Authority, although some children went along to the specially converted school wards for some classes. These children usually made their own way across to the schoolrooms, unsupervised.

Only the very youngest children in the two homes remained in their cottages during school hours. Over half the children in both homes went to nursery or primary schools within the grounds of the establishments, and these were the last to leave for school. Older children went to secondary schools outside the homes, or to work, and many of them travelled long distances by public transport. These children got themselves ready for school, subject to a quick check by the housemother, and it was usual for older children to supervise the younger ones on their way to school—as would children in a normal family. In all four establishments, children returned to their living units for lunch at midday (except for some of those attending secondary school outside the homes, who took school dinners).

One of the major activities in all establishments on at least some days each week was bathing. In most places, this was done in the afternoons, after the children had returned from school. All children in the subnormality hospital were bathed at least three times a week: many were bathed daily, and some of the severely incontinent had to be bathed more frequently still. In this hospital, bathing was usually carried out immediately the children had been toileted, following afternoon tea. This meant that the bathing period often lasted until after 6 p.m. when the wards had fewest staff on duty. Because of this, in about half the wards, all of the children were kept in the bathroom from the time toileting began until the whole toilet–bathing routine was completed. The children were then put to bed. In other wards, children were taken to their beds in the dormitory immediately they had been bathed, to avoid the problem of supervising active children in the dayroom. Only three of the high-grade wards returned some of the children to the dayroom to play before they went to bed, and for the rest there was little recreational activity when bathing was in progress. During bathing itself, in nine of the wards the staff organized themselves on the conveyor-belt system already discussed.

Bathing was usually done in the mornings in the paediatric hospital, at a time when more staff were available. Even so, three out of the five wards used a conveyor-belt system in the bathroom. Many of the children who were severely handicapped, however, were bathed on their beds each day, and given a 'proper' bath only once a week.

About a third of the children in the homes required supervision or assistance in bathing, but this was always done individually: in only one of the fifty-eight separate cottages investigated was anything like the conveyor-belt system in operation. In all the remaining cottages, bath-times provided an opportunity for individual contact between staff and children. The children would normally be playing indoors or outside until their turn for the bathroom came round. Afterwards, except for the youngest children, they could sit around and watch television or play games before they went to bed. All of the children had at least two baths a week as required by Home Office regulations, though many had more frequent baths than this. Although bathing was usually done in the early evenings, children could bath at other convenient times, with permission.

It has already been mentioned that the children in the hospitals got up remarkably early. Not surprisingly, many of them went to bed while the sun was still high in the sky, at weekends as well as on weekdays. In one ward of each hospital, bed-time for the youngest children started at 4 p.m. and in nearly half the wards it had started by 5 p.m. In five subnormal wards and one paediatric ward, bed-time was between 6 and 7 p.m., and in the three highest-grade subnormality wards and one paediatric ward, a few children were allowed to stay up until 8 p.m. They did not, however, sleep undisturbed. In most of the wards in both hospitals the children were potted at intervals throughout the night. It was common for nearly all of them to be lifted three times; a few children could be checked as many as five times during the night, to see if they were wet or dirty. It was not uncommon for all children in the ward to be potted, whether or not they wet their beds, if the night nurse was new to the ward.

Bed-times during the week in the children's homes varied from 6.30 p.m. to 10 p.m. Each housemother decided on bed-times for the children in each cottage, and, not surprisingly, older ones stayed up later than younger ones. At weekends children could stay up later still. Many of the younger children took toys to bed with them, while the older ones read until 'lights out'. On several occasions, staff were observed reading stories to the younger children in bed, although this was never observed in the hospitals. Little, if any, potting was done at night. Houseparents usually lifted known bed-wetters last thing at night, before they themselves went to bed.

There were many other ways in which the lives of the children in the two kinds of establishment differed. All children in the two homes had their own clothing in adequate, if not over-plentiful, supply. Most of them had some choice in what they wore, usually by going with the housemother to make purchases, and some of the older children could buy their own clothes from their clothing allowance. Virtually all of them had their own toys, and most had their own books, as well as the communal toys provided for each cottage. Although, as has been mentioned in Chapter 5, the living units were short of individualized storage space, nearly all of the children had somewhere to keep their own possessions to which no one else had access. They used such places to the full, storing many treasured possessions. In the subnormality hospital, the only item which was provided by the institution for all children was a toothbrush: 87 per cent had shoes, 75 per cent had overcoats, 35 per cent had slippers and 15 per cent had combs or hairbrushes provided by the hospital for their own use. None had underwear, shirts, blouses, trousers, skirts, jumpers, cardigans, dressing gowns, pyjamas or handkerchiefs which had been provided by the hospital and which they could call their own. Instead, each child was dressed from a central supply of clothes, according to approximate size. The clothes were not named, and once sent back to the laundry they were not returned to the same child. A few children had private clothes supplied by parents and which were kept for special occasions, but there was little storage space for clothes of this kind and the practice was not encouraged. It was not unusual for wards to run out of clothes of a particular size, so that the children were often to be seen wearing ill-fitting garments. Some wards attempted to stockpile clothes to avoid this problem. The children had few toys or books of their own, and although nearly all of them had bedside lockers, the lockers were used only at night to store clothes for the next day—so that the night nurse knew what to dress them in the next morning. Often lockers were used to store excess bedclothes. On more than half the wards, toys were kept locked in cupboards in the dayroom, or else placed tidily on ledges which were out of reach of the children. In the paediatric hospital things were better, and the bedside lockers were filled with many personal items. But even here, only just over half the children had their own jumpers or cardigans, and only one child in four had a shirt or blouse, whether supplied by the hospital or by parents.

There was a good deal more freedom in the cottages of the homes than there was in the wards. Children could use the gardens and the grounds more or less as they wished, and there were few places which were out of bounds. They mostly had the run of the house, although some housemothers imposed more restrictions than others. In most cottages, the children had spent some time at least in the staff quarters. They could bring paintings home from school and have them hung on the walls of their bedrooms. Treatment too, for the most part, was adapted to the child's age and maturity. All of the children received pocket money which was distributed by the housemother. The amount varied according to age, and children were encouraged to save to buy things they wanted. When they had saved enough, the housemother would go with them to make the purchase. The children were permitted to go to other cottages to play and to have tea, and could, in return, bring their friends back to their cottage. Birthdays were special occasions, on which the birthday child received cards, a small present and a birthday tea. There was a full range of clubs and activities to occupy the time in the evenings and at weekends.

The world of the children in the hospitals was much more restricted: inside the units they were limited to the dayroom and the sanitary annexe during the day, and the dormitory at night: they were rarely allowed to use the kitchen, and sister's office was out of bounds. Outside the unit the children in the subnormality hospital could use the courtyards only under supervision, and the hospital grounds only when escorted to and from school, or the zoo, or when taken on 'a walk'. Children in the paediatric hospital had, in theory, rather more freedom, but few were able to use it because of their handicaps. As a result, one of the remarkable things about the hospitals, to a visitor, was how few of the children were to be seen outside, even in fine weather. Only the school-children in the subnormality hospital received pocket money, although 'children' in the paediatric hospital over the age of sixteen received a weekly sum from the National Assistance Board. It was rare for the children in either hospital to be taken to outside shops by the members of staff. In both hospitals there was a marked lack of contact between children in different wards except when they were at school; visiting another ward for a meal hardly occurred at all. One consequence of this was that when a child was moved from one ward to another, which happened frequently, he might never again see either the staff or the children in his old ward except fortuitously. Most wards in the subnormality hospital attempted to provide 'jellies and other extras' for tea when a child had a birthday, but only if the child was thought 'likely to benefit', and no presents were provided by the establishments.

It was evident from the field study that children in the paediatric wards had a somewhat less bleak existence than those in the mental subnormality hospital, but that even pre-school children in the children's home were likely to enjoy more personal freedom, and to receive more individual attention than any of the children or adolescents in either hospital.

We hope we have not given the impression, in a short account of this kind, that there were no difficulties for staff and children in the homes. In most cottages there were examples of petty restrictions surrounding certain aspects of life, and inevitably there were clashes of personality and differences of opinion from time to time. The point is that these were the exception rather than the rule, and that, in contrast to the hospitals, the cottages provided a system of care geared very closely to the individual needs of those for whom it existed. It should not be thought, on the other hand, that the nursing staff in the hospitals were in any way deliberately unkind in their treatment of the children, or neglectful of their duties. At no time did we see treatment which could be placed in these categories. In any case, the patterns of care were so similar throughout the wards within each hospital that the existence of particular child management practices could not be accounted for by the behaviour or attitudes of individuals. Other factors needed to be considered in accounting for the different systems of care in the different establishments.

## A replication study

One possible explanation for the differences in the systems of care could be sought in the differences between the handicaps and abilities of the children. It could be argued that the patterns of care found in the homes were simply not attainable with children so disabled as those in the hospitals, or even that the handicaps of the hospital children in some sense necessitated the particular patterns of management adopted. Neither view seemed to us an adequate explanation: other studies (e.g. Tizard, 1964), have shown that it is possible to bring up severely retarded children in residential care in a manner which resembles that found in the best residential nurseries; and some schools for children with severe physical handicaps are run in a manner which offers a rich, varied and seemingly satisfying environment. To obtain further comparative evidence about child upbringing in residential institutions for the handicapped, however, the two sociologists conducted additional studies in two rather different establishments serving the needs of severely retarded children (King and Raynes, 1968b). The research procedures used were identical to those adopted in the homes and hospitals.

One of these establishments was a voluntary home for the severely subnormal organized by a private society. The institution had extensive and pleasant grounds in an isolated, rural area. It housed seventy-six inmates in all, who were accommodated in several buildings: adolescent boys and girls lived with housemothers in new, detached cottages; younger children lived in an old mansion known as 'the school'; there was also a special care unit for children with severe physical handicaps, which was staffed, in part at least, by trained nurses. The other establishment was a small hostel for the severely subnormal, administered by the mental health department of a Local Authority. The hostel was a detached, purpose-built unit on the edge of a council housing estate. Close by was a day training centre run by the same Local Authority, to which the children in the hostel, as well as others from the community, went on a daily basis.

The regimen in these institutions was very different from that already found in the subnormality hospital. Yet many of the children in the hospital closely resembled those in the hostel and the voluntary home in terms of age, IQ and severity of handicap Indeed, one high-grade ward in the hospital and one unit in the voluntary home contained children who were so similar in these respects to those in the hostel, that the comparison of their régimes provides a test of the hypothesis that children's handicaps necessitate one régime rather than another.

## Three groups of severely subnormal children

The ward contained eighteen children, the hostel sixteen children, and the unit in the voluntary home twenty-two children. Each of the groups had a majority of children between the ages of seven and twelve years. The differences between the mean ages of the three groups were not statistically significant, and the age distribution is given in Table 7.1.

TABLE 7.1  *Percentage age composition of three groups of severely subnormal children*

|  |  | N | Birth to 6 years | 7–12 years | Over 13 years | No inf. |
|---|---|---|---|---|---|---|
| Ward | Mean age 12y. 2m. | 18 | 0 | 67 | 33 | 0 |
|  | SD        1y. 6m. |  |  |  |  |  |
| Hostel | Mean age 11y. 11m. | 16 | 6 | 50 | 44 | 0 |
|  | SD        3y. 6m. |  |  |  |  |  |
| Voluntary home | Mean age 11y. 5m. | 22 | 5 | 64 | 27 | 5 |
|  | SD        2y. 8m. |  |  |  |  |  |

The majority of children in each of the groups were imbeciles with IQs in the range 21–50 points. Again, the mean differences between the groups were not statistically significant, and the percentage distribution of children in different intelligence categories is given in Table 7.2.

All children in each of the three groups were able to walk without the help of the staff or assistance from mechanical aids.

## The hospital ward

At the risk of some repetition, it will be useful to describe a typical day in this ward for comparison with the two other units. Ward accommodation comprises a large dormitory, a smaller combined dayroom and diningroom, a treatment room and bathroom and toilets for the children. In addition, there is a staff office, a kitchen, and a small, separate cloakroom for the staff. A fenced playground is shared with the adjacent ward. The ward is staffed

TABLE 7.2   *Percentage distribution of intelligence in three groups of severely subnormal children*

| | | N | Idiots (IQ 0–20) | Imbeciles (IQ 21–50) | Feeble-Minded (IQ 51+) | No. inf. |
|---|---|---|---|---|---|---|
| Ward | Mean IQ 31.0 | 18 | 0·0 | 88·0 | 6·0 | 6·0 |
| | SD 10·4 | | | | | |
| Hostel | Mean IQ 37·0 | 16 | 12·5 | 75·0 | 12·5 | 0·0 |
| | SD 14·0 | | | | | |
| Voluntary home | Mean IQ 36·0 | 22 | 9·0 | 68·0 | 14·0 | 9·0 |
| | SD 14·6 | | | | | |

by nurses working a shift system. On a typical day there would be a charge nurse and two student or assistant nurses on duty from 7.30 a.m. until 2 p.m. A different charge nurse and two different junior nurses would take over the ward until 7.30 p.m., overlapping with the morning shift from 1.30 p.m. until 2 p.m. One member of staff would go off duty at 6 p.m., leaving two staff members on the ward between 6 p.m. and 7.30 p.m. None of the staff are resident in the unit and from 7.30 p.m. until 7.30 a.m. the day staff is replaced by one night nurse. Most main meals are cooked off the ward in central kitchens. Domestic duties are performed by domestic staff who are allocated to serve two or more wards.

The children sleep in one large dormitory. The beds are lined along each side wall. The dormitory is brightly painted but sparsely furnished. The counterpanes on each bed are identical. Each child has a bedside locker in which are kept blankets and other ward equipment. The clothes the child is to wear on the following day are also placed there. The walls are not bare of pictures, but those which can be seen are far above the eye-level of the tallest child.

The day begins at 5 a.m., when all the children are awakened by the night nurse. She takes them as a group to the toilet. There, all eighteen children are sat on chamber pots or toilets in the bathroom. After toileting they are washed and brought back to the dormitory. Some children go back to sleep, while others lie awake in their beds. At 6 a.m. the night nurse begins to dress the children, working her way round the ward. Because there is little time, and some of the children are slow at dressing, many who could dress themselves are, in fact, dressed by the night nurse.

By 6.45 a.m. most of the children are dressed and sitting on the floor of the dormitory. When the children are dressed, the night nurse makes the beds. Just before the day staff arrive at 7.30 a.m., the night nurse sits the children on the ends of their beds. She is now ready to hand over the ward.

The children are taken by the day staff into the dayroom as one large group, where they sit at small tables while the staff prepare the breakfast. The radio, situated high on the wall, is switched on by the staff. The television set is kept locked away in a wall cupboard. Breakfast is served just after 8 a.m. and is finished by 8.30 a.m. The children are again taken as one group to the toilets. One member of staff supervises the toileting, while another supervises hand-washing, teeth-cleaning and hair-combing. The charge nurse is in the office during this time. The children leave the bathroom individually and congregate in the passage outside, where they can be seen by the charge nurse from the office. Here they wait until all have finished in the bathroom, when they go for a few minutes to the dayroom, which has been cleaned after breakfast. They do not stay there long, because sixteen of the children attend the hospital school full-time, for two hours in the morning and two hours in the afternoon. At 9.10 a.m., a nurse supervises the putting-on of topcoats and then takes the children to the school in the hospital grounds. The two children remaining in the ward are left alone, while staff check the laundry and clean the treatment room. Only occasionally do staff have any contact with the children.

The schoolchildren return at 11.45 a.m. and are toileted immediately on their return. Lunch is delivered from the central kitchens between 11.45 and 12.15. The children are seated at the tables for some time before the meal is served. As for all other meals, the children sit three or four to a table. A trolley is wheeled into the room and the staff serve the food from there to each table in turn. Each child is given just the plate of food and a spoon or a knife and fork. Apart from this, the plastic-surfaced tables are bare. None of the staff ever sit down to eat with the children, and since all but one of the children feed themselves, staff supervise from a position by the trolley, replacing one plate by another when necessary. An occasional remark of reproof or approbation about a child's eating habits constitutes the sum total of conversation during the meal. The meal is messy. All of the children have bibs or aprons tied around them for each meal. After lunch, the children wait at the tables 'to allow their dinners to go down'. Then they are again taken to the toilet. By 1.15 p.m. the schoolchildren are ready to leave for the afternoon session. Again, the two children remaining on the ward are left to their own devices.

After school, the children return to the ward and are toileted before tea, which begins at 4 p.m. After tea, bathing begins. Because the dayroom is once again being cleaned, the children are all taken to the dormitory where they sit and play on their beds. From there they are taken, two at a time, to the bathroom. There, one nurse baths the children while another dries and dresses them. The charge nurse meanwhile supervises the children in the dormitory. When the children have all been bathed they are taken into the dayroom, which has now been cleared, for playtime. This occurs at about 5.30 p.m. Sometimes the children play with a variety of small toys, and occasionally the staff join in with a quiet game. More often this time is spent watching the television, which is unlocked by the charge nurse. The youngest children leave for bed at 6 p.m. The older ones stay up until 7.15 p.m. They are toileted before being put to bed for the night, and the ward is then handed over to the night nurse. During the night, some of the incontinent children are wakened again at midnight and at 2 a.m. for toileting.

This régime is changed only slightly at weekends or during the school holidays. Getting-up times, bed-times, toilet-times, bath-times and meal-times do not vary very much throughout the year. Even at weekends it is only in the afternoons that time is found for the children to play in the yard outside, and then only in the finest weather. Occasionally they are also taken for walks in the grounds or down to the football field.

None of the children have free access to the kitchen, the dormitory, the office or indeed to any part of the ward. Although the doors are not kept locked, children are not encouraged to enter any of these rooms except under supervision or for specific purposes such as doctors' visits. Few of the children have possessions or toys of their own, and none has a complete set of clothes which is kept for his personal use. Instead, toys quickly become communal property, and clothes are distributed daily, according to approximate size, upon their receipt from the laundry.

*The Local Authority hostel*

On the ground floor of the hostel there is a diningroom, a playroom, a kitchen, a utility room, an airing room and toilets and cloakroom for the children. In addition, there is a self-contained flat for the superintendent and a staff toilet and wash basin. Upstairs, there are half-a-dozen small bedrooms, some with wash basins, for the children, and two bathrooms and toilets. A sickroom and accommodation for the resident housemother are also situated on the first floor. Surrounding the hostel are lawns, the front one giving direct access to the road.

On a typical day, the unit is staffed by either the superintendent or her deputy, the resident housemother, who work from 7 a.m. until 9 p.m., with two hours off-duty taken in the afternoon. In addition there will be one or two assistant housemothers who are on duty while the children are in the hostel. At night, the hostel is looked after by one of two housemothers (one of these is the only member of staff who is nursing trained), while the resident will be 'on call'. Cooking for the unit is done by a part-time cook who comes in for all meals, except midday during the week, while the children are out. Four part-time domestic staff look after the cleaning of the hostel and complete the establishment. This staffing of the unit is supplemented by students and other voluntary helpers from the community who come in to play with the children.

The children sleep in small bedrooms with two to four children in each. The bedrooms are bright and cheerful and are decorated in different styles. The children have space in their rooms for personal possessions and clothing. Some of the children have put pictures or photographs of their families around the rooms, which contribute to their individual character.

The children are wakened during the week between 7 a.m. and 7.15 a.m. and many of them begin to get themselves up, washed and dressed—some of them wash in their rooms. The night nurse goes round giving assistance to those who need it, and the resident comes upstairs to wish the children 'good morning'. As soon as they are washed and dressed, the children begin to filter downstairs to the dayroom, where they look at comics, play, or listen to records, which they choose and operate for themselves. One of the older children remains upstairs and helps with the bedmaking before she comes down for breakfast. The two oldest boys take their breakfast as soon as they are ready, and the resident walks with them to the door to see them off when the coach calls to take them to an Industrial Training Unit. For the remainder of the children, breakfast begins at about 8.30 and lasts until about 9 a.m. After breakfast, all the children have to go to the toilet, but they go individually, and apart from four who require some assistance, they take themselves. They wash and comb their hair, the superintendent or her assistant checking to see that the job has been done properly. Before they leave for the day training centre across the road, accompanied by a member of the hostel staff, there is usually time for a song or some 'back-chat'.

During weekdays, the children are away from the hostel until the end of the afternoon session at the training centre. The staff consequently use this period to get on with necessary chores around the unit and also to take their periods of off-duty. The main meal of the day takes place in the evening, after the children have returned. They get back to the hostel at about 3.15 p.m. and take their coats and outdoor shoes off. These they put away in the cloakroom. Each child has his own peg and individual locker. In the latter, the children keep some of the bits and pieces which they bring back to the hostel from the training centre. Before tea, the children play and talk with one another and members of the staff in the dayroom.

The children go into the dining-room for tea at about 4.30 p.m. The two tables there are each laid for nine or ten persons. The tables are covered with tablecloths and there is a place set for each child. Plates of bread and butter and cakes are also on the table. At one end of each table are a teapot and cups and saucers. Here a member of staff sits, eating with the children—as is the case at all other meals in the hostel. The children say a short grace and the cook brings in the food from the kitchen. There is continuous chatter throughout the meal with staff and children talking to each other. The plates of bread and butter and cakes are passed up and down the table as required. Food is kept hot for the two older boys who return later than the others, and they join in the meal as soon as they arrive. The meal, which lasts about an hour, is regarded by all as an important social occasion. At the end of the meal, the superintendent indicates to the children at one table that they must get down and go to the toilet and then to the playroom. The children at the remaining table help to clear away the tea things before they too go to the toilet and then join the others.

In the playroom after tea, staff, children and any visiting helpers join together in a variety of activities. The children put records on the record player, and the housemother gets up to dance with two or three children. Some children rush about boisterously in play; others concentrate on jigsaw puzzles or painting. Staff are constantly chatting with the children and can be seen reading to them. The staff make a point of engaging the interest of as many children as possible, and a considerable range of social relationships are sustained. Play activities continue whilst some of the children are bathed.

One member of staff baths the boys; another baths the girls. While the bath is running, the child collects his pyjamas from his room and goes for his bath. He is returned to the playroom while the water is left running for the next bath, and so the process goes on. The youngest children are put to bed by 7 p.m. while the older ones stay up until about 8.30 p.m. The superintendent helps with putting the children to bed, and she says prayers with the children in each bedroom before tucking them in for the night.

At weekends, the routine is very different. Some of the children go home at weekends, but those who stay have a 'lie in' in the morning and go to bed later at night. They take all their meals with the staff, sometimes in the superintendent's apartment, which is an integral part of the building. Much of the weekend is spent in play outdoors and in visits to local shops and places of interest. On Thursday evenings some of the children go to a local club for handicapped children.

There are a number of restrictions placed upon the use of the rooms in the hostel, but all of the children use the rooms at some time, and to some, such as the airing room, they have free access for play at odd times without supervision. All of them spend some of their time in the sittingroom of the superintendent's flat. All of the children possess their own individual clothing which is marked with their name. They know and recognize which are their own clothes and toys and which of them belong to other children. The whole régime, in fact, is remarkably similar to that found in the cottages of the children's homes of the original study.

## The voluntary home

This group of children has physically the poorest accommodation. They are housed in an old, rambling building which is scheduled to be replaced. Accommodation is on two floors. The bedrooms are not so well furnished as those in the hostel, but the children's drawings and picture postcards are stuck up on the walls. Also upstairs are a playroom, a medicine room and a sewing room, and an office as well as toilets and bathrooms for the children, and a flat for the resident matron. Downstairs are three classrooms, a kitchen, a diningroom, more bathrooms and toilets, and a staff sittingroom. On a normal day, the unit is staffed by the matron (who is on call virtually throughout the week) and four assistant housemothers, who are given responsibility for special groups of children, and who are off-duty during school hours. In addition, three schoolteachers come to the unit every morning and afternoon during the week, and also on Saturday mornings. A part-time cook comes in to prepare most of the meals, although the midday meal is prepared in a central kitchen and sent over in containers to the unit. There are three part-time domestic staff who do the cleaning.

The general pattern of everyday activities and child-care practices resembles that found in the hostel, although there are some differences. Here, the children go to school actually in the same building. The children are bathed and toileted individually. Meal-times, as in the hostel, are occasions in which both staff and children participate. There are five tables; the matron and head teacher sit at one and children and assistant housemothers sit together at the others. The tables are laid with knives and forks and glasses. The meal is served at the tables by the assistant house-mothers. There is much conversation between staff and children throughout the course of the meal, which is ended by the matron calling a child to say grace. After this, the children stand up, clasp the hands of their neighbours and, turning to them, say 'thank you'. The matron then indicates which table should lead out first and as the children pass her, she speaks to each of them in turn. Playtime, which is after tea, is spent by the children with their housemothers either in their own bedrooms or in the playroom, which the groups take turns in using. Staff join in with the children's games.

All of the children have personal clothing, marked with their names, and most of them have toys of their own.

In a few respects, however, the régime resembles that in the hospital ward. Before breakfast, the children are grouped together and wait for a bell to ring, which is the signal to go downstairs. After lunch, there is a 'quiet period', in which some of the children are encouraged to lie down for half an hour before afternoon activities begin. There is also some lack of flexibility of the routine from one day to another, and not all of the children are permitted access to all of the available living space in the unit.

## Summary

In this chapter we have described the main elements in the systems of care and management in six institutions, based on our observations in all of the separate living units, as well as interview data collected from the head of each unit.

It was evident that the two children's homes were very similar to each other in their régimes, and very different from either of the two hospitals. Life in the paediatric hospital, however, was somewhat less rigid and devoid of interest than that in the subnormality hospital. It seemed unlikely that differences in the handicaps of the children could have accounted for the different patterns of care, and some confirmation of this was found when two further institutions for the retarded were examined. Two groups of children were identified who were very similar to those in one of the high-grade subnormality wards. One of these groups, in a Local Authority hostel, enjoyed a way of life very like that found in the children's homes; the other, in a voluntary home, was managed in a way which shared some of the hospital and some of the hostel characteristics.

In the next chapter, we try to present these differences in systematic quantitative terms, and discuss some preliminary conclusions.

# 8 Child management: some preliminary conclusions

The account given in Chapter 7 of the ways in which children in different types of institution spend their day suggests that what they do, and what they are allowed to do, are influenced by factors other than the handicaps of the children. Indeed, the similarity among all the living units within each institution, and the wide differences between types of institution, suggest that institutions develop their own distinctive norms of child management. Our later enquiries explored in more detail relations between organizational and structural factors in the different institutions and the environment open to the children living in them. Before undertaking further studies, however, we attempted to make more objective, and to express in quantitative terms, the differences we had already observed in child upbringing patterns.

In this we took as our starting point the work of Goffman. The value of Goffman's (1961) essay on total institutions, already discussed in Chapter 4, was that it pointed to functional similarities between types of institution which differ radically both in the characteristics of their inmates and in the ostensible purpose which they serve. In our studies, for example, both hospitals approached the 'ideal type' of a total institution; the children's homes and the two smaller units for mentally retarded children described in the previous chapter do not. However, it was evident that none of the institutions was as 'total' as a concentration camp or an old-fashioned asylum; the paediatric hospital was less total than the mental subnormality hospital; and the voluntary home for subnormal children was more total than the Local Authority hostel. The dichotomous classification of total or not total was therefore too crude for analytical purposes, and the next step was to quantify the differences between the institutions, to express them on a scale or scales representing continua or dimensions along which they varied.

Goffman's account of total institutions incorporates a description of staff–staff interaction as well as inmate–inmate interaction, but much the most significant part of his analysis from our point of view is concerned with the points of contact between the staff and inmate worlds. We have attempted to operationalize aspects of staff–inmate interaction along what we have termed the dimension of *inmate management,* or more specifically, *child management.*\*

All the features of staff–inmate interaction, or inmate management, which Goffman describes as characteristic of the total institution may be regarded as having a common orientation in that they pay scant regard to the individual differences among inmates or to changes in circumstances which may occur from time to time. Because of the special nature of people-work in institutions, according to Goffman, the points of contact between the staff and inmate worlds involve 'a constant conflict between humane standards on the one hand and institutional efficiency on the other' (1961, p. 78). In the examples Goffman cites—the design of garments, the distribution and laundering of clothes, the management of hair-cutting and so on—this conflict is usually resolved 'in favour of efficiency' and 'the smooth running of an institutional operation' (p. 79). In our early thinking, we were inclined to accept that many of the management practices in institutions were, in fact, geared to efficient institutional functioning and the convenience of the staff, as Goffman suggests. As our studies progressed, however, it became apparent that some practices, while they certainly denied the individuality of the inmates, were neither particularly convenient for the staff, nor necessarily efficient. Thus, the conveyor-belt system of washing and toileting a large group of children at the same time, which was employed by many of the hospital wards described in the previous chapter, actually created more problems of supervision than would have been involved had one member of staff kept the children occupied in the dayroom while another took them one at a time to the toilets. Nonetheless, in their

---

\* Although our measures relate to the management of children, much the same considerations would be involved in the management of adults in other types of institutions. It should be noted that Goffman was undecided about the status of 'orphanages' as total institutions. He included them in his denotative list (1961, p. 4), but eight pages later he considered excluding them from the category. This was because he sees total institutions as forcing houses for changing the self, and because children, in their capacity as 'not-yet-persons', have no fully developed self to change. Goffman's logic here seems to us to be faulty – presumably even an incomplete self can be changed under the influence of institutional living. To push his argument to extremes, one would have to exclude mental hospitals on the ground that the self-concept of the mental patient is already distorted by his illness: but to do this would be to destroy much of what has been most illuminating in Goffman's work.

105

systematic denial of individuality, the kind of management practices discussed by Goffman do seem to represent one end of a continuum or dimension of possible management practices. For want of a better term, bearing in mind the above remarks, we have called practices of this kind *institutionally-oriented practices*. At the other end of this continuum one may expect to find practices where individual differences among inmates and unique circumstances are given recognition by the institutional staff, and where variations in routine are tolerated or encouraged. Such practices we describe as *inmate-*or *child-oriented management practices*.

In attempting to operationalize this conceptual dimension in children's institutions, we concentrated on four areas of child management and staff–child interaction: the rigidity of routine; 'block treatment' of children; depersonalization of children; and the social distance maintained between children and staff. The polarity between *institution-orientation* and *child-orientation* in each of these areas is discussed below.

### Rigidity of routine

Management practices are institutionally-oriented when they are inflexible from one day to the next and from one inmate to another. Individuals in different situations are treated as though they were in the same situation, and changes in circumstances are not taken into account. Management practices are child-oriented when they are flexible, being adapted to take into account individual differences among the children or different circumstances. Thus, for example, one may attempt to discover whether management practices are characterized by rigidity or its absence by asking questions about the time children get up and go to bed, and by establishing whether these times are unchanged throughout the week or not. One may also ask, as we did, about the existence of set times at which the children can use their bedrooms, or the garden, and about times at which their parents may visit them.

### 'Block treatment'

Child management practices are institutionally-oriented if the children are regimented—that is, all dealt with as a group—before, during or after any specific activity. These practices involve queueing and waiting around, with large groups of other children and with no mode of occupation during the waiting period. Such regimentation we describe as 'block treatment'. Management practices may be described as child-oriented where the organization of activity is such that residents are allowed to participate or not, as they please, and when they are allowed to do things at their own pace. For example, one may ascertain whether children are 'block treated' on getting up, before or after bathing, at the toilet, before and after meals, and so on.

## Depersonalization

Child management practices may be seen as institutionally-oriented when there are no opportunities for residents to have personal possessions or personal privacy. Depersonalization is also shown when there is an absence of opportunities for self-expression, or of situations in which initiative on the part of the children may be shown. Where there are opportunities for residents to show initiative, to have personal possessions, to be alone if they so desire, the child management practices may be described as child-oriented. For example, one can examine what is done with the personal possessions the children bring with them to an institution. It is also possible to find out if, after admission, the children are allowed to retain any clothing or toys of their own, and if there are places in which they can keep these.

## Social distance between children and staff

Management practices are institutionally-oriented when there is a sharp separation between the staff and inmate worlds. This may be because separate areas of accommodation are kept for the exclusive use of staff, or because interaction between staff and children is limited to formal and functionally specific activities. Child orientation involves the reduction of social distance by the sharing of living space, and allows staff and children to interact in functionally diffuse and informal situations. The degree of social distance between staff and children can be assessed by finding out, for example, whether staff eat with the children, or watch television with them, or whether the children have access to all rooms in the cottage or ward in which they live.

## The construction of a Child Management Scale

In seeking items which might form the basis for a Child Management Scale, we decided to limit ourselves to factual items which referred to everyday *practices,* and for which a high degree of reliability could be expected, rather than items which attempted to measure staff opinions, or which referred to hypothetical or rarely occurring events. We discarded items which relied for their validity on any particular theory of child development, and instead sought to devise items which could be applied in a range of institutions

107

but which provided objective indications of the four categories of management practices listed above. We tried to avoid items which might be dependent on cultural norms, or the age, intelligence or handicaps of the children, as far as this was possible. Many items which appeared to be relevant to child management, and some which clearly differentiated between institutions, failed to meet these criteria and were therefore discarded. For example, items relating to the management of food fads, and the practice of permitting children to read in bed, were dropped from the list because they were dependent on age and handicap, as well as cultural factors. Some items, the response to which could be a function of a child's ability to walk, were for this reason asked only of ambulant children.

Following initial pilot work, a large number of items of information which appeared to meet the criteria was collected in each of the institutions. The information was collected by use of an interview schedule (see Form B1, p. 218) which was administered to the person in charge of each living unit. Selected items from this schedule made up the Child Management Scale. Questions were related to specific situations occurring on the day the interview took place, and as far as possible to specific children randomly selected from within each unit. In this way it was hoped to avoid generalized responses and thus increase their validity. Observations were carried out in each unit, close to the day of interview, to verify those responses which could be validated by observation. Of the items which could be validated by cross-checking, no difference was found between item scores based on observations and those based on interview data. The reliability of the information was assessed—by comparing responses elicited by two interviewers from the same interviewees, and by comparing the observation schedules recorded by two observers at the same time —and both interviews and observations were found to be reliable. The level of agreement between interviews was 94·2 per cent and between observations was 92 per cent (Raynes and King, 1968).

The response to each item was scored on a three-point rating scale. A score of 0 was given if the response indicated child-orientation, while a score of 2 indicated institution-orientation. Where the pattern revealed a mixture of institution-orientation and child-orientation, a score of 1 was recorded. Items which could not be unambiguously scored in this way with a high degree of agreement between raters were discarded.

An item anaylsis was carried out to test for discrimination and linearity, and only those items which met the criteria recommended by Maxwell (1961) were retained to form the Child Management Scale.

In our early studies, where we had to restrict our items to those which related to comparable areas of child management practice in homes for the deprived as well as institutions for the subnormal, a scale was developed which consisted of sixteen items. As each item could be scored 0, 1 or 2, the range of possible scores was 0 to 32. In later studies, which were confined to institutions for the retarded, it was possible to reintroduce more items. One item was dropped from the original scale and a further fifteen items were added, so that the revised scale had a range of possible scores from 0 to 60. The correlation between the new items and the old, for sixteen institutions studied in our later survey, was $r = 0.92$. Table 8.1 lists the items in each of the areas of the revised scale. A fuller account of the development of the original scale has been given by King and Raynes (1968a); the revised scale is given in full in Appendix I together with the scoring categories, and some information about its construction and properties.

It is important to note that the preparation of the original scale was carried out *before* any observations were made in the voluntary home or the Local Authority hostel. Thus, while the original scale was to some extent constructed in such a way as to reflect differences we had already observed between the two hospitals on the one hand and the two children's homes on the other, the scale itself was applied as it stood to the voluntary home and the Local Authority hostel, neither of which had been contacted until work on the scale had been completed.

## The use of the Child Management Scale in six institutions

Striking differences were found in Child Management Scale scores between the four large institutions. The two children's homes had a range of scores from 0–5 and 0–6 respectively. The paediatric hospital had a range of scores from 17–22, and the mental subnormality hospital a range from 23–30.

There was no difference between the mean institution scores obtained from the twenty-two cottages in the first home and from the thirty-six cottages in the second home. Both of these scores were significantly different from the scores obtained from the five wards of the paediatric hospital ($p < 0.001$). There was also a highly significant difference between the mean score of wards in the paediatric hospital and those of the mental subnormality hospital ($p < 0.001$). The data are given in Table 8.2.

The scores for the two children's homes indicate a high level of child-oriented practices. By contrast, the subnormality hospital reflects a high level of institutionally-oriented practices, and although the score obtained by the paediatric hospital falls into an

TABLE 8.1   *Revised Child Management Scale items*[a]

*Rigidity*

1 (AC)* Do children get up at same time at weekends?
2 (AC)* Do children go to bed at same time at weekends?
3 (AC)* Do they use the yard or garden at set times?
4 (AC)* Do they use their bedrooms at set times?
5        Are there set times when visitors can come to visit?
6        Which children are routinely toileted at night?

*'Block treatment'*

7 (AC)   After dressing do children wait around doing nothing?
8 (AC)*  Do they wait in line before coming in for breakfast?
9 (AC)*  Do they wait together as a group before bathing?
10 (AC)* Do they wait together as a group after bathing?
11 (AC)  How do they return from the toilets?
12 (AC)  Do they wait at tables before the meal is served?
13 (AC)* Do they wait at tables after meals before next activity?
14 (AC)  How are they organized for walks? ·

*Depersonalization*

15   What is done with their private clothing?
16   What is done with their private toys?
17*  How many possess the following articles of clothing?
18*  Whereabouts do they keep their daily clothes?
19*  How many have toys or books of their own?
20   Do they have pictures, photos, etc. in their rooms?
21   How much time do the children have for playing?
22   How are children's birthdays celebrated?
23   How are tables laid for meals?

*Social distance*

24 (AC)* Do the children have any access to the kitchen?
25 (AC)* Do the children have any access to other areas?
26       How do staff assist children at toilet times?
27*      How do staff assist children at bath-times?
28*      Do staff on duty eat with the children?
29       Do staff sit and watch television with children?
30 (AC)  How many children have been on outings with staff?

---

[a]Items marked * were items asked on original Child Management Scale – see King and Raynes (1968a). Items marked (AC) relate to ambulant children only. For fuller details on methods of scoring, sources of data and item analysis, see Appendix I.

intermediate position on the scale, it lies much closer to the sub-normality hospital than to either of the two homes.

An examination of the mean scores obtained by the institutions on each of the groups of items relating to *rigidity, 'block treatment', depersonalization,* and *social distance* shows that management

TABLE 8.2   *Child Management Scale scores in four establishments*

| Establishment | Mean | Standard deviation |
|---|---|---|
| First home | 2·41 | 2·89 |
| Second home | 1·43 | 1·46 |
| Subnormality hospital | 26·07 | 2·63 |
| Paediatric hospital | 19·60 | 2·07 |

Values of '$t$'
  1st home and S.S.N. hospital $t = 24·55$, $p < 0·001$
  2nd home and S.S.N. hospital $t = 44·67$, $p < 0·001$
  1st home and paediatric hospital $t = 19·87$, $p < 0·001$
  2nd home and paediatric hospital $t = 23·91$, $p < 0·001$
  S.S.N. hospital and paediatric hospital $t = 8·81$, $p < 0·001$

practices in the children's homes were in each case child-oriented, while those in the hospitals were institutionally-oriented. The only area in which there was a significant difference ($p < 0·01$) between the mean scores of the first and second children's homes is that of *depersonalization.* There were statistically significant differences between the two hospitals in *rigidity* ($p < 0·02$) and *depersonalization* ($p < 0·001$), the paediatric hospital being in both cases somewhat less institutionally-oriented in its practices than the subnormality hospital. The differences between the hospitals and the children's homes in each of these four areas were very highly significant statistically. Table 8.3 gives the data.

Although there was a range of scores of eight points in fifteen wards of the subnormality hospital (one ward could not be scored because it contained no ambulant children), the evidence did not support the view that it was the wards with the largest numbers of severely handicapped patients in which the most institutionally-oriented practices were found. It will be recalled from Chapter 5 that six wards accounted for 65 per cent of all the profoundly retarded children (IQ 0–20), and 69 per cent of the children who were least able to walk, as well as a high proportion of those with other management problems. Of these wards, two were among the four highest scoring units, that is, the most institutionally-oriented, and two were among the four lowest scoring or child-oriented units.

The replication study gave little support to this view, either. The scale was applied in exactly the same way in the Local Authority hostel and in all the units of the voluntary home. In the previous chapter, we gave a detailed description of the routines in one of the hospital wards, the Local Authority hostel and one of the units in the voluntary home, all of which contained children

TABLE 8.3 *Child Management Scale scores in rigidity, 'block treatment', depersonalization and social distance: four establishments*

| Establishment | Rigidity | | 'Block treatment' | | Depersonal- ization | | Social distance | |
|---|---|---|---|---|---|---|---|---|
| | (Mean) | (SD) | (Mean) | (SD) | (Mean) | (SD) | (Mean) | (SD) |
| First home | 0·77 | 1·11 | 0·05 | 0·68 | 1·05 | 1·25 | 0·55 | 0·80 |
| Second home | 0·94 | 1·30 | 0·00 | 0·00 | 0·43 | 0·56 | 0·06 | 0·20 |
| Subnormality hospital | 7·06 | 0·71 | 5·73 | 1·58 | 7·47 | 0·92 | 5·80 | 1·52 |
| Paediatric hospital | 6·00 | 0·71 | 4·40 | 1·14 | 3·00 | 2·21 | 6·20 | 1·07 |

In an earlier publication, King and Raynes (1968a), the scores in some institutions for depersonalization and social distance were unfortunately transposed.

similar in their age, sex, intelligence and handicaps. Table 8.4 gives the scores for these units on the Child Management Scale.

TABLE 8.4    *Child Management Scale scores for three groups of severely subnormal children*

|  | Rigidity | 'Block treatment' | Deperson- alization | Social distance | Total scale |
|---|---|---|---|---|---|
| Ward | 7 | 7 | 8 | 8 | 30 |
| Hostel | 3 | 2 | 1 | 0 | 6 |
| Voluntary home | 6 | 3 | 0 | 2 | 11 |

As can be seen from Table 8.4, the hostel caring for subnormal children falls within the range of scores attained by cottages in the two homes caring for normal but deprived children. The unit in the voluntary home scored less than half the score of the most child-orientated ward in the subnormality hostel. Another unit in the voluntary home, the special care unit, cared for children who were as severely handicapped, mentally and physically, as any of those in the hospitals. This unit scored 14 points on the scale, 8 less than any ward in the subnormality hospital and 3 less than

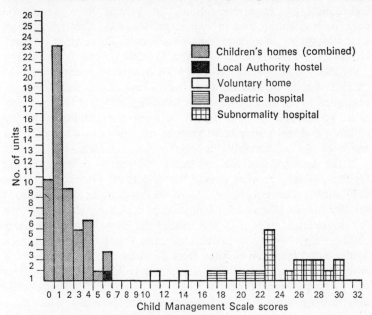

Fig. 8.1 *Distribution of scores for six institutions*

any ward in the paediatric hospital. The remaining units in the voluntary home, all of which cared for a mixture of mildly and severely subnormal young adults, obtained a mean score of 3·7, which was well within the range of the children's homes.

Fig. 8.1, which presents all these findings graphically, brings out the differences in total Child Management Scale scores between units in the various institutions. The data, especially those obtained from the hostel and the voluntary home, gave us confidence that the scale did, in fact, provide a quantitative measure which would enable different institutions to be compared. The scale was sufficiently sensitive to reflect the degrees of difference between the patterns of care already described in Chaper 7. The revised scale of thirty items, used in the studies described in Part Three, provided an even more effective and discriminating instrument.

## Discussion and preliminary conclusions

The field studies described in this and the preceding three chapters have indicated a wide range of variation in institutional upbringing in establishments caring for normal and handicapped children. Institutionally-oriented child management practices were found in both the hospital for subnormal children and in a hospital for children of normal intelligence who had chronic and severe physical handicaps. Deprived children of normal intelligence who were in residential care in two large, longstay children's homes were brought up in a manner which was much more child-oriented. However, severely retarded children, brought up in a hostel and in a voluntary home, were also cared for in a child-oriented manner, so that the differences between institutions could not simply be attributed to the differences in the handicaps of the children. Moreover, no association was found between the handicaps of the children and the management patterns of their units when different wards of the subnormality hospital were examined.

If the handicaps of the children could not be held to account for the differences, what could? There was no evidence from the field studies that either the size of the institutions or the size of the living units played any significant part. Among the institutions for the retarded, it is true, the smaller the establishment the more child-oriented were the patterns of care; but both the children's homes cared for more children than the subnormality hospital, and without exception their living units were child-oriented. The sizes of living units were so similar in all establishments that they could not possibly explain the differences in care patterns. What these data appear to show is that large institutions are not necessarily bleak and barren places, and that small living units in themselves provide no guarantee of child-oriented patterns of care.

There was similarly no evidence to suggest that child-oriented units were better staffed, or that their staff had received more training, than institutionally-oriented units. Indeed, when ratios of *assigned staff* were compared for the different establishments in Chapter 6, the institutionally-oriented units in the two hospitals were better staffed than the child-oriented units in the children's homes. However, although the homes had fewer staff, they worked longer hours and their duty periods were arranged so that the fit between staff availability and the demands of the children's routine was more efficient. When *effective staff ratios* were compared, therefore, the differences between establishments in assigned staff were offset. It is difficult to make straightforward comparisons, however, because at some times of day the units in all establishments were better staffed than at others. The staffing patterns in the hostel and the voluntary home for the subnormal resembled those for the children's homes. Obviously, adequate numbers of staff are desirable to maintain good standards of care: but even units which are greatly stretched in terms of staffing can be successful in providing child-oriented practices. The institutionally-oriented practices in the hospitals were not due to shortages of staff, and it seems that the allocation of adequate staff alone does little to ensure a child-oriented pattern of management. A higher proportion of nursing staff had received training for their work, and over longer periods, than child-care staff in the other institutions, so the *fact* of training is unlikely to provide an explanation for the pattern of care.

Our data thus suggested that the handicaps of the children, the size of institutions and living units, the staff–child ratios and the proportion of staff who were trained were not decisive factors in influencing child management practices. Instead, the reasons for the differences seemed to lie partly in the *kind* of training the staff received, and partly in the way in which the establishments, and especially the units within establishments, were organized. It was these factors which appeared to limit what the staff could do, and to govern the way in which they performed their roles.

We did not examine the content of staff training courses in any detail, although it seems probable that some forms of training are more appropriate than others, and the kind of training received may well influence staff towards one pattern of care more than another.

The organizational features which appeared to be most closely related to child-oriented patterns of care and management may most conveniently be considered under the general concept of 'household organization'. Goffman (1961, pp. 11–12) pointed to the incompatibility between family life and the total institution; and argued that the maintenance and strengthening of households in the community provided the best form of resistance against the encroachment of the total institution. What he apparently did not consider was the possibility that some institutions may deliberately organize themselves in the form of households or quasi-households.

The child-oriented units in all establishments shared certain factors reminiscent of family households in the community. Indeed, it had long been the policy of the children's homes, following the Curtis Report, to establish units run on 'family group' lines, and the hostel and voluntary home for the subnormal followed very much in this tradition. Staff worked in the units on a stable and permanent basis, without being required to move from one unit to another, and with some staff, at least, resident in the unit. Children, too, in such units, were not required to move in the course of their stay in the establishment. Staff of all grades shared in the activities of the unit, as would the members of a normal family, without a marked division of labour between junior and senior staff. The persons in charge of such units were given some responsibility for budgeting the household expenditure, and for buying clothes and toys for the children: and for the most part they were trusted to get on with it. But they could also be found cooking, mending and looking after the everyday needs of the children.

In the institutionally-oriented hospital units, none of these features was present. Both staff and children were moved from unit to unit, and there were noticeable differences in the roles of different grades of staff. The wards appeared to function as rather tightly controlled units with little responsibility delegated to the sisters or charge nurses, who were regularly supervised by senior members of the nursing administration. Sisters in turn delegated little responsibility. It seemed likely that this system of organization imposed strict limits on the variation in patterns of care which could be tolerated between units, and also militated against the personalized treatment of the children. If each ward had a similar routine, which was not dependent upon the unique characteristics of the children within it, then it could more easily assimilate the frequent changes of staff. If tasks such as cooking, buying clothes, laundering and mending were performed by centralized agencies outside the units, staff working in the units were less likely to feel an overall responsibility for events. If the organization of the ward took little account of individual differences among the children, unit staff were less likely to be aware of them either.

These speculations formed the starting point for the survey, reported in Part III, which was designed to explore more systematically the relations between organizational variables and child management in institutions for the subnormal. But before leaving the field studies, a word should be said about the possible effects of different patterns of care on the children who experience them.

It was not possible, of course, in these studies to draw any conclusions about the effects of different patterns of care. Statements about these could follow only from a different research design which included data collected on a longitudinal basis. However, there was some evidence to suggest that in institutions with child-oriented management practices, subnormal children were more advanced in feeding and speech than their counterparts in institutionally-oriented establishments. The results of a comparison between the three groups of severely subnormal children described in Chapter 7 are consistent with the findings of earlier experimental studies.

It will be recalled that the three groups of children were similar in age, intelligence and physical handicaps. All the children were described by staff as being able to feed themselves, with the exception of one child in the ward, who had to be fed. The ways in which the children were able to perform this activity, however, were very different, as is shown in Table 8.5. The superiority of the home and hostel children over the ward children is marked

TABLE 8.5   *Feeding skills of three groups of severely subnormal children (%)*

| | N | Use knife and fork | Use spoon | Have to be fed |
|---|---|---|---|---|
| Ward | 18 | 11 | 83 | 6 |
| Hostel | 16 | 94 | 6 | 0 |
| Voluntary home | 22 | 91 | 9 | 0 |

and highly significant statistically ($p < 0.001$). Again, the ward children were noticeably more backward, with regard to speech, when compared with the home and hostel children. Once more, the differences are statistically significant ($p < 0.02$).

It seemed possible that these differences could be directly attributed to certain characteristics of the management practices in each institution. In the hostel and the home, meal-times were social occasions in which the staff joined the children to eat: the children were given encouragement to develop their skills and had adult role models to follow. In the ward, meals and their administration were part of the work-load for the staff. Sometimes children who

TABLE 8.6  *Verbal skills of three groups of severely subnormal children* (%)

| | N | Use sentences | Use isolated words | No intelligible speech |
|---|---|---|---|---|
| Ward | 18 | 17 | 39 | 44 |
| Hostel | 16 | 56 | 25 | 19 |
| Voluntary home | 22 | 45 | 27 | 27 |

could feed themselves were fed by staff in order to speed the process up. Since staff never ate with children, there were no adults on whom to model their meal-time behaviour. As to the speech differences, it was very noticeable that staff spoke to children more frequently in the hostel and the home than in the ward. Moreover, much of the talk which did occur in the ward consisted of giving instructions rather than friendly 'chat'. These observations made it seem worth while to try to measure the frequency and warmth of staff–child interactions, and particularly the frequency of talking to children, in our later studies.

**part three**


# Some determinants of care: A survey

# 9 Child management practices and institutional organization: some hypotheses

The field studies reported in Part II were followed by a more systematic survey carried out in sixteen institutions, all of which cared for severely retarded children. Most severely subnormal children requiring residential care in the country are accommodated in one of three types of institutions: hospitals under the National Health Service, hostels under the Mental Health Departments of the Local Authorities, and homes run by voluntary societies, many of which have a number of contractual beds paid for by the Health Service. We studied units in five hospitals, eight hostels and three voluntary homes.

The study was designed to throw more light on some of the organizational factors which appear to influence patterns of child management as these are measured by the revised Child Management Scale. Before describing the research design and methods of study, which we do in the next chapter, the aims of the investigation will be set out here in the form of a series of hypotheses. It can be seen that the hypotheses arise directly from the earlier studies.

Our first four hypotheses are concerned with the broad administrative categories which the institutions represent, the characteristics of their inmates, and the size of the institutions and their constituent units.

## Hypothesis 1

That large and characteristic differences in child management practices will be found between the three types of institutions caring for severely subnormal children.

121

*Hypothesis II*

Although in extreme cases particular handicapping conditions may require particular modes of treatment, in general the differences found in management patterns will not be related to the level of handicaps of the residents.

*Hypothesis III*

Differences in the child management practices of different living units will not be related to the overall size of the establishments in which the units are found.

*Hypothesis IV*

Nor, within the broad limits expected to be found in this country, will child management practices be related to the size of the constituent living units themselves.

The next three hypotheses are concerned with aspects of staffing the living units:

*Hypothesis V*

Obviously, there are limits below which staffing cannot be allowed to fall if child-oriented management practices are to be maintained. On the other hand, the provision of many staff is no guarantee that institutionally-oriented practices will not occur. Within the limits expected by current British standards in units for children, therefore, child management practices will not be related to the ratios of *assigned* staff to children in the living units.

But child-care practices will be related to staffing in two ways:

*Hypothesis VI*

Units which are characterized by child-oriented patterns of care will organize their staff duty arrangements so that most staff are on duty at times when there are most children in the living unit. In institutionally-oriented units, numbers of staff on duty at particular times will not be related to the numbers of children in the unit, or the nature of the activities, at those times. That is, whatever the *assigned staff ratios*, child-oriented units will be characterized by better *effective staff ratios*.

*Hypothesis VII*

In units which are child-oriented in their management practices, there will be greater continuity of staff, and smaller staff turnover, than in institutionally-oriented units. The latter will be characterized by frequent changes of staff for reasons unrelated to the needs of the children (e.g. because there are staff shortages elsewhere, or so that students can 'gain experience' by working in different units, and so on).

In our conclusions to the field studies, we put forward the view that child-oriented units shared many features of what might be called 'household organization' whereas institutionally-oriented units did not. From this general position a number of more specific hypotheses have been derived.

### Hypothesis VIII

The role activities of senior staff will be systematically related to the patterns of child management in the following way. In units with child-oriented patterns of care, the head of the unit will spend a higher proportion of her activities involved in the social and physical care and supervision of the children than the heads of institutionally-oriented units. The latter will spend a greater proportion of their activities on administrative or domestic duties which will not bring them into direct contact with the children.

### Hypothesis IX

The heads of child-oriented units, whatever the nature of their role activities, will spend a greater proportion of their time in the presence of children than the heads of institutionally-oriented units. Moreover, when they are with them, their interaction will be characterized by more warmth and a greater frequency of talk, than will be the case for the heads of institutionally-oriented units. That is to say, the ways in which unit heads *perform* their roles will be related to the scores on the revised Child Management Scale.

### Hypothesis X

There will be more diffusion of role activities as between senior and junior staff in child-oriented units, and greater specificity of role activities as between senior and junior staff in institutionally-oriented units. That is to say, when the activities of different grades of staff are compared, there will be greater similarities between grades in the child-oriented units than in the institutionally-oriented units.

### Hypothesis XI

Junior staff in child-oriented units will, like their seniors, interact with the children in a way characterized by greater warmth and a greater frequency of talk than their counterparts in institutionally-oriented units.

### Hypothesis XII

The activities of heads of units within the unit will be related to the amount of responsibility they are given within the wider organization of the institution. Heads will be *more* involved in personal child care when they have a personal responsibility for *more* aspects of the unit's functioning, than when they are 'relieved' of such duties and responsibilities. The amount of responsibility given to the head of the unit, or the unit autonomy, as we have called it, can be measured in several ways. Specifically, we expect the heads of units who are most involved in physical and social child care and supervision of the children will also have most autonomy and responsibility as evidenced by:

(1) greater freedom from inspection and supervision by superiors;
(2) greater control over child-care decisions;
(3) greater control over decisions relating to buying goods for the children and for the unit;
(4) greater control over staffing decisions; and
(5) greater control over matters of unit management.

Our final hypothesis was concerned with the training of unit heads and the possible effects of this on the way they performed their roles and the management practices in their units.

### Hypothesis XIII

The role performance of unit heads—that is, the way in which they carry out their duties as measured by the frequency and warmth of their interaction with the children, and especially the frequency of talking—will be related to the training they have received. We expect the unit heads who have high rates of interaction with the children will have had a training in 'child-care', in which such matters are given some emphasis: unit heads with low rates of interaction are more likely to have received a nurse training in which there is a primary emphasis on the physical aspects of health and disease. It follows from our earlier hypotheses that we also expected the units with 'child-care' trained heads to be more child-oriented in their management patterns than the units with nurse-trained heads.

It is difficult to see how any single piece of research, undertaken at one point in time, could do equal justice to all these hypotheses. Our study was, of necessity, a cross-sectional survey and this design has inevitably served us better in relation to some hypotheses than to others.

We have tried to point out where our findings must be regarded as more tentative, but for most hypotheses we have been able to accumulate systematic evidence. Obviously, it has not been possible in a study of this kind to explore the effects of different management patterns on the children who experience them. This would have required data collected longitudinally, or on an experimental basis. Where we have collected data in this area, we have reported the findings, although these cannot be regarded as a test of any relationship between patterns of care and the development of children. We hope that this list will have given a clear indication of the nature of our later enquiries, and that it will serve as a reference point in reading the subsequent chapters.

Hypotheses I to IV are discussed in Chapter 11; V to VII in Chapter 12; VIII to XI in Chapter 13; and XII and XIII in Chapter 14.

# 10  Research design and methods

Sixteen establishments for the severely subnormal were selected for our survey. Eight of these were Local Authority hostels for children; five were mental deficiency hospitals within the National Health Service which cared mostly for retarded adults but which also had some wards for children; and there were voluntary homes which took some patients under contractual arrangements with Regional Hospital Boards as well as private patients.

A number of factors entered into the selection process. Limited time and money meant that only sixteen institutions could reasonably be studied and that these should be conveniently accessible from London. Within these limits we wished to find institutions from the three main types of provision which would enable us to explore further the hypotheses set out in the previous chapter. As far as possible we wanted to study establishments of different sizes within each institutional type. The hostels were selected at random, with a proviso that half should contain fewer than 20 patients, from a list of hostels obtained from the Ministry of Health. The smaller hostels contained 12, 15, 16 and 19 children respectively: the larger ones had 21, 23, 23 and 41 children. The hospitals were all much larger than the hostels, but there were very big differences in size among them: they contained 121, 380, 1,007, 1,457 and 1,650 patients respectively. The voluntary homes were a heterogeneous trio of intermediate size, larger than the hostels but smaller than any of the hospitals, with 50, 83 and 93 children in them. The hospitals and voluntary homes were selected largely on the basis of geographical convenience, and we do not suggest they are necessarily representative of hospital or voluntary home provision in this country. In a study of this kind, however, we were less concerned with the generality of our findings than in exploring the nature of the relationship between certain variables and the patterns of care, and the choice seemed adequate for this purpose.

The centre of interest in this study was once again the living units in which the children were accommodated. Seven of the eight hostels contained only one major living unit. In the hospitals, the voluntary homes and the remaining hostels, where there were several separate units, we selected only one from each establishment for inclusion in the study.

In order to reduce the variance between living units as far as possible it was decided to select units in which all, or nearly all, the children were ambulant, severely subnormal and between the ages of five and sixteen years. Since no published data about the units within any of the institutions were available, it was not possible to make this selection until after a discussion was held with the medical superintendent or warden on the arrival of the research worker. From the information he gave us, we then selected the unit in the establishment which most nearly met our criteria. The living units selected in this way varied in size, the hostels having from eight to forty-one residents and the hospitals from twenty-seven to forty-seven. There were ten, twelve and eighteen children in the units selected in the voluntary homes. For convenient reference in the tables and text we have numbered the hostels from 1 to 8, and lettered the hospitals A to E. The three voluntary homes are referred to as X, Y and Z.

The establishments and their living units varied greatly in physical layout. Of the eight local authority hostels, two (hostels 2 and 3) were old houses which had been converted to their present use, and six were new, purpose-built dwellings. Five of the latter provided accommodation on a five-day-week basis, with some provision for weekend care, while the other three hostels provided full-time care. All were adjacent to, or a short distance from, a Local Authority training centre which was attended by mentally retarded children living in their hown homes as well as by the residents living in the hostels. In general, the hostel accommodation was of a high standard, having separate sittingrooms, dining-rooms and kitchens, small bedrooms sleeping from one to four children, and an adequate number of bathrooms and toilets which were convenient to use. They also had a sluice room, sometimes a sickroom and sewing room, a laundry, and a staff flat or flats for senior, and sometimes junior, staff. They were well furnished, with adequate cupboards and wardrobes, as well as individual lockers for children. All were situated in their own grounds with yards and gardens for the children to play in. Most were in or near the centre of towns.

In their physical provision, the hospitals presented an unfavourable contrast to the hostels, four having been built before the First World War. Although all had been much modified and upgraded since the introduction of the National Health Service, they all showed their age and had an institutional look about them. One was situated on the outskirts of the city, and four were in rural areas fairly close to small towns.

Two of the hospital wards we studied had only a single dayroom which also served as a diningroom; another had two dayrooms, while two had three separate dayrooms which were also used as diningrooms. The dormitory accommodation was, in all cases, subdivided. One ward had two bedrooms for six children, one bedroom for four children, one for nine and three single bedrooms, only one of the latter being occupied at the time of the research. The remaining wards all had larger dormitories with between twelve and twenty-five beds. All the hospital units had their own kitchens and staff offices, courtyards and playing areas. Each was part of a larger establishment set in extensive grounds. Their institutional appearance was due not so much to a general shortage of space, as to the fact that, because of the age and design of the buildings, much of the space could not be used to best advantage. There was also a comparative absence of toys, pictures and personal possessions in the rooms, in some units a lack of curtains, and in all a lack of the homeliness which characterized the children's hostels. Accommodation for some staff was provided in separate buildings, away from the children's living units, but within the grounds of the hospitals.

The three voluntary homes were all in rural areas. One had formerly been an old hall, while the other two were large converted houses that had been added to. They were all sub-divided into a number of separate living units. In the first unit we studied, the children were accommodated in three four-bedded rooms which were also used as dayrooms, although the children went to a central diningroom for meals. In the second, the children lived, slept and ate in one large room with eighteen cots. The third unit had ten children sleeping in one room, where they also spent their days, except for meals which were taken elsewhere. In one unit the children were provided with lockers, and toilet and other personal possessions were in evidence. Such things were not to be seen in the other two units. Accommodation was provided for most of the staff in living units separated from the children's but within the grounds of the establishment. Two of the voluntary homes (Y and Z) had much the poorest accommodation of any of the units we visited. All were inconvenient places, and the toilet facilities in particular were unsatisfactory, but they all had large grounds. In organizational structure, with several loosely integrated units, they were intermediate between the hospitals and the hostels. (A fuller description of the institutions has been given by Raynes, 1968.)

## The children

The characteristics of the residents in the different establishments are listed in Table 10.1 together with the total scores on the revised Child Management Scale.

Eighty-five per cent of the children were aged between 5 and 16 years. On average they were slightly older than the children in the field studies, the mean age being $11\frac{1}{2}$ years. Of the 190 children in the five wards, only 2 were less than 5 years of age, but 42 were aged 16 or more, 38 of these being in two hospitals. Of the 162 children in the hostels, only 2 were less than 5 years of age and 7 more than 16 years. The children in the voluntary homes were a younger group, 10 out of the 40 being less than 5 years of age, while no child was aged over 14 years. The hospital children as a group (mean age 12 years 11 months) were significantly older than the hostel children (mean age 10 years 11 months), who were, in turn, significantly older than the children in the voluntary homes (mean age 7 years 8 months). All the hostels had children of both sexes, whereas two hospital wards (wards B and D) were for boys only and one ward (ward A) was for girls. Voluntary home X had only girls and voluntary home Y had only boys. In all, boys made up 54 per cent of the hostel population, 68 per cent of the hospital group and 62 per cent of the children in the voluntary homes.

The classification of children by grade of mental retardation for the three types of institution is given in Table 10.2. In the hospitals and the hostels, about one child in every six or seven was unclassified, but two-thirds of the remainder were severely retarded children with IQs ranging from 20 to 50 points. The hospital wards contained twenty-seven children (14 per cent) who were classified as being profoundly retarded or idiots, whereas the hostels had only five (3 per cent) of such children. The large proportion (40 per cent) of children who were unclassified in the voluntary homes makes the data here difficult to interpret.

One-third of the children in the hostels (34 per cent) and in the voluntary homes (32 per cent) suffered from Down's syndrome, as compared with only a quarter of the children in the hospitals (27 per cent).

We have already said that we attempted to select units in which the majority of children were ambulant. As Table 10.1 shows,

129

TABLE 10.1 Characteristics of residents in sixteen units by type and size of establishment, size of unit and revised Child Management Scale score[a]

| Type of establishment | Total size (children) | Unit size (children) | Mean age years | Percentages with IQs 0–20 | 21–50 | 51+ | Unknown | Percentage mongols | Percentage ambulant | Revised Child Management Scale scores |
|---|---|---|---|---|---|---|---|---|---|---|
| **Hostels** | | | | | | | | | | |
| 1 | 23 | 23 | 11·2 | 0 | 65 | 21 | 13 | 22 | 100 | 10 |
| 2 | 41 | 41 | 11·3 | 3 | 66 | 12 | 19 | 41 | 95 | 6 |
| 3 | 21 | 21 | 8·6 | 14 | 67 | 5 | 14 | 52 | 100 | 14 |
| 4 | 16 | 8 | 12·6 | 0 | 12 | 0 | 88 | 63 | 100 | 4 |
| 5 | 19 | 19 | 10·8 | 0 | 84 | 16 | 0 | 32 | 95 | 22 |
| 6 | 15 | 15 | 10·5 | 7 | 67 | 13 | 13 | 27 | 94 | 3 |
| 7 | 12 | 12 | 10·6 | 0 | 92 | 0 | 8 | 42 | 100 | 18 |
| 8 | 23 | 23 | 11·6 | 0 | 78 | 13 | 9 | 9 | 100 | 11 |
| **Hospitals** | | | | | | | | | | |
| A | 380 | 32 | 15·5 | 16 | 62 | 9 | 13 | 25 | 78 | 47 |
| B | 1,457 | 44 | 12·9 | 7 | 75 | 4 | 14 | 36 | 98 | 37 |
| C | 1,650 | 41 | 12·3 | 24 | 61 | 22 | 12 | 15 | 95 | 45 |
| D | 121 | 26 | 8·3 | 23 | 73 | 0 | 4 | 42 | 92 | 45 |
| E | 1,007 | 47 | 14·3 | 6 | 68 | 2 | 23 | 21 | 100 | 41 |
| **Voluntary homes** | | | | | | | | | | |
| X | 83 | 12 | 9·2 | 17 | 67 | 8 | 8 | 58 | 83 | 14 |
| Y | 93 | 18 | 5·2 | 6 | 17 | 0 | 78 | 22 | 11 | 41 |
| Z | 50 | 10 | 10·2 | 20 | 60 | 10 | 10 | 20 | 90 | 28 |

[a]Percentages rounded to nearest whole number.

TABLE 10.2 *Percentage distribution of children by intelligence categories*[a]

| Type of institution | Idiots (IQ 0–20) | Imbeciles (IQ 21–50) | Feeble-minded IQ 51+ | IQ not known | No. of children |
|---|---|---|---|---|---|
| Hostels | 3 | 69 | 12 | 16 | 162 |
| Hospitals | 14 | 68 | 4 | 14 | 190 |
| Voluntary homes | 12 | 43 | 5 | 40 | 40 |

[a]Figures rounded to nearest whole number.

more than 90 per cent of all children in all but three establishments were fully ambulant, and most of the remainder could, in fact, crawl or shuffle or walk with assistance. In hospital A, 12·5 per cent of the children required assistance in walking and 9·4 per cent were bedfast or had to be carried, which meant that 78 per cent were fully ambulant: in voluntary home X, 83 per cent were ambulant and 17 per cent required assistance. The one institution which did not have mostly ambulant children was voluntary home Y, in which only 11 per cent were able to walk unaided. This home was, in several respects different from all the other units in the study. It is difficult, therefore, to treat the voluntary homes as a group and for some analyses they have been omitted. There was no statistically significant difference, however, between the hospitals and the hostels in the proportions of ambulant children which they had.

Few children in any establishment had serious deficiency of sight or hearing. Epilepsy was, however, reported somewhat more frequently. A significantly higher proportion of hospital children than hostel children suffered from epilepsy: fifty-one hospital children (27 per cent), as opposed to twenty-seven hostel children (13 per cent). The proportion in the voluntary homes was higher still, being 30 per cent (twelve children out of forty, in the units studied). But there were few children in any of the units who suffered from cerebral palsy or other physical defects, and no group of institutions was significantly worse than the others in these respects.

Other differences between children in the three types of institution will be discussed in later chapters. The data given here show, however, that though the hostels contained a far from negligible proportion of children who were severely handicapped, hospital wards contained still more. The interpretation of any differences in child management practices or other aspects of unit life is complicated by these differences in the characteristics of the resident population, as well as by the differences in the size of the establishments and the units. However, some units from institutions of different types can be matched on several variables, and some comparisons can be made among institutions of the same type.

Our efforts at matching the children in terms of their age and ability to walk were not as successful as we should have liked. However, in the absence of published data on the basis of which we could have selected units prior to obtaining permission to visit and study them, there was little else to do but make the best of the situation we found on arrival. (To have attempted to obtain the data on size of living units and the characteristics of inmates in advance, would have constituted a research project in itself.) None the less, we do not think that the differences in age composition, proportions of ambulant children, or, indeed, any of the other differences between the populations, were sufficiently large to account for the differences we found in child management by themselves.

## Procedure

Permission to undertake the investigation was first obtained from the senior administrative officer or Medical Superintendent of the establishment. None of those who were approached refused his permission. The purpose of the enquiry was outlined in general terms, and both at this point, and every later stage in the investigation, we answered all questions fully and honestly.

A member of the research team spent a period of five days in each of the living units studied. On arrival, he introduced himself to each staff member of the ward or unit, and the purposes and methods of procedure for the study were outlined. Questions were always invited, and if staff seemed at any stage in the investigation to be troubled by the presence of an investigator, further discussions were held at which questions were again invited. Times were arranged for interviews and for observations. Staff were assured of the confidentiality of all the information collected during the enquiry, and this promise was kept.

Data were collected on the children, their management, and the activities of the staff. Some of the schedules used had been developed in the field studies. These were revised in the light of experience and, together with certain new instruments, were extensively piloted in four other organizations before we undertook the survey: two residential nurseries for normal children, one hostel for the retarded and one mental deficiency hospital. Particular attention was paid at this stage to the assessment of the reliability of the instruments, and three fieldworkers were involved in all the reliability studies. Reliabilities of all the instruments used in the final studies were found to be very high, and any techniques which did not meet our criteria of reliability were abandoned. For observation techniques, where it seemed that reliability might decline over a period, further checks were made towards the end of the survey. In fact, reliability remained as high at the end as it had been at the beginning. The instruments are discussed briefly below, and are reproduced in full, together with details of how they were tested, in the Appendices.

## Information about children

This was recorded on two schedules, Form A1 and Form A2, which are shown in Appendix II (p. 214). The data were obtained partly from case records, kept either in the unit or in a central office, by the fieldworkers themselves who completed Form A1; and partly from the senior member of the unit staff through a questionnaire, Form A2. The head of each unit was left with one copy of the A2 schedule for each child in the unit. These were to be returned to the research unit in a pre-paid envelope, after the research worker left. The fieldworker always went through one form in detail with the unit head, and then left the remaining forms in a folder, which also contained a set of definitions and instructions. The unit heads were most co-operative. All of them returned all of the schedules fully completed for every child in their units.

Schedules A1 and A2 provided us with the information about the child's age, his date of admission to the institution and to his present unit, the number of other units he had lived in, his clinical diagnosis, grade of defect, and other physical handicaps (epilepsy, sensory handicaps, ability to walk). Questions were asked about each child's skills in feeding, dressing, speech and toilet. Other questions (taken from Kushlick [personal communication]) were asked about over-activity, agressiveness, attention-seeking behaviour, destructiveness, self-injury, running away, tantrums and withdrawal or solitariness. In the third section of Form A2, questions were asked about how often the children were visited, and by whom, and about their personal clothing.

## Child management practices

The thirty items in the revised Child Management Scale have been reported in Chapter 8 (pp. 107–14) and are presented in more detail in Appendix I. The scale was scored partly on the basis of observation and partly from what we were told at an interview with the head of each unit. Form B1 (pp. 218–21) was used to record the interview data. It is a detailed interview schedule, designed to elicit information about how the children in the units spent their time throughout a typical weekday and during the weekends. As far as possible, questions were made to refer to what had happened on the *previous day,* but the staff were also asked whether this was a typical day or whether there were variations in the routine. Staff were also asked about children's clothes and toys, and about where they kept personal possessions, about whether they could go into the dormitory or kitchen as they wished, about going outside, walks, going out of the grounds, having friends in to tea or to play, about the arrangements for children's birthdays, and about going home.

Responses to some of these questions were checked, using an observation check list (Form B2, pp. 231–3), and additional observations were made on this schedule of the management of situations which were more readily observable than asked about.

## Staff activities

Data were obtained on these in several ways: interviews, recording schedules completed by staff and returned to the research unit after the fieldwork, and observations.

### Interview and recording schedules

With the help of the staff, three schedules were completed on staff activities. The first of these (Form C1, p. 221), provided a detailed time-table of the hours during which all the staff were working on the unit for the week of the fieldwork. This was obtained on the first day of the research worker's visit to the unit, to enable him to plan his observational studies, and was then checked again at the end of the week, so that any staff changes that might have occurred could be noted. This form was used in the calculation of staff ratios. The unit organization schedule (Form C3, p. 223), which was used in an interview with the head of the unit, gave us information about the way in which the unit was organized.

We obtained from this the number of part-time and full-time staff and whether they were resident or not. We enquired about 'family grouping', whether special responsibilities were given to particular staff members, and about how decisions regarding purchases of clothes and toys for the children were made, how birthday presents were obtained, and about what arrangements were made for the children's holidays. We asked whether the head of the unit had a petty cash allowance, and if so, what it was used for. A further set of questions related to decisions regarding the children; for example, how they were admitted to the unit, whether or not they should attend school, whether or not they should go home, and so on. Other questions asked how decisions affecting the deployment of staff were made, whether there were regulations from superiors regarding the running of the unit, and how often the unit was visited by a person of higher authority. Nine questions were asked, following a technique effectively used by Coser (1962), which were designed to investigate staff attitudes to the unit, but the information obtained from these, although interesting, did not lend itself to quantitative treatment.

Before the investigator left the unit, a questionnaire (Form C4, p. 227) was given to all staff members, who were asked to fill it in and return it to the research unit in a stamped, addressed envelope which was provided. This gave us information about the sex, age, marital status and the number of children staff members had, their social class (as measured by their father's occupation), and some details of their work in the establishment. A response rate of 85 per cent was obtained for this questionnaire.

Finally, we conducted a simple interview with the head of the establishment as a whole. This provided us with information about the number and size of the constituent units, and the general administration of the establishment.

## Time-sampling observations

Observations which, in aggregate, amounted to nearly two full days of observing and recording were made on a time-sampling basis. They were designed to provide us with detailed information on the activities of the staff and the way in which they interacted with the children in their care. The observations were organized as follows: staff were first divided into three broad grades—the head of the unit; junior child-care or nursing staff; and domestic staff. Each grade was observed for a period of three minutes, in such a way that thirty seconds of observation were followed by thirty seconds of recording. After the third period of recording observations in the three-minute period, there was a two-minute interval during which the observer located the next person to be observed. In each fifteen-minute period the head of the unit was observed first, then a member of the junior nursing or child-care staff, and finally a member of the domestic staff was studied. As a rule, there was more than one junior staff member on duty at one time, and sometimes more than one domestic. The order in which junior staff and domestics were observed was determined from a prearranged, random sequence, once it was known (from Form C1) which staff would be on duty.

The observers used a recording schedule, Form C2 (p. 233), and a stop-watch. Each page of the recording schedule represented a fifteen-minute period, and therefore enabled us to complete one full cycle of observations for each of the three grades of staff. The observations were carried out from the time the children got up until they went to school or, where some children did not go to school, until 10.30 a.m. If there were children not attending school, additional observations were carried out for one hour at midday and for a further hour in the early afternoon, using the same technique. Then, observations were carried out from the time the children came back from school, or, where the children were not at school during the day, from 4 p.m. until the children had been put to bed, or until 8 p.m., whichever was the earlier. Observations were spread over a period of four days and two periods of afternoon observations and two periods of morning observations were included in every unit, to reduce the risk that we were watching an atypical situation.

It would be idle to pretend that staff and children were unaware of the fieldworkers' presence; but surprisingly few difficulties were encountered, even in the initial phases of observation. The fieldworkers went to some lengths to explain that it was not a 'time and motion study', and that they were not concerned with 'efficiency'. Everybody in the units had to get on with the business of the day, whether fieldworkers were present or not, and staff very quickly settled down to an apparently normal pattern of work. It soon became possible for the observer to move about the units, carrying recording schedule and stop-watch, in a reasonably unobtrusive manner.

The observations were tested in the four pilot institutions over many weeks by three observers. The time interval of thirty seconds was decided after many different intervals had been tried and rejected. After much experimentation, the final form of the schedule was devised so that only a minimum of recording was required of the fieldworker. The following data were collected during the observation periods:

(1) The activities performed by the member of the role group being observed;
(2) The interaction, physical and verbal, between staff and children;
(3) The location of the activity and the number of children present at the time.

Activities of the staff were classified in five categories: administrative, domestic, supervisory, physical child-care (e.g. bathing, dressing, feeding the children), and social child-care (which involved staff in educational and recreational activities with the children). Each category was denotatively defined by a check list of activities, which had been developed during the pilot studies, and a coding system was devised for recording purposes. The categories proved, in the event, very nearly exhaustive, and a sixth classification, miscellaneous, rarely had to be used. A brief description of the activities was also recorded, so that the accuracy of coding could subsequently be checked in the office. In each thirty-second interval of observation, we also recorded whether or not the observed member of staff spoke to any of the children. No record was made of the content, tone or duration of their conversation, because no reliable way of doing this could be found during the pilot study. The reliability of the observations was extremely high and full details are given in Appendix III (pp. 233–44).

In the following chapters, some of the data yielded by these instruments are presented, in so far as they relate to the hypotheses already outlined.

K

# 11 Child management practices in hostels, hospitals and voluntary homes

In the last chapter, we described briefly the institutions we studied in the survey. They differed in organizational type and size, as well as the kind of accommodation they provided for the children in their care. The children themselves, although mostly ambulant and of school age, differed in a number of respects. It is now our task to examine the relationship between these variables and the patterns of child management used in bringing up the children. We provide no further descriptive material on child management: instead, we use the scores on the revised thirty-item Child Management Scale as our index of the patterns of care. Here we examine the first four hypotheses which were presented in Chapter 9.

*Hypothesis 1*

The first hypothesis (p. 121) stated that we should expect to find large and characteristic differences between institutions of different types in which retarded children were accommodated. The scores of the revised Child Management Scale which were assigned to each unit clearly substantiate this hypothesis.

The revised Child Management Scale scores, calculated for each of the sixteen units, ranged from 3 to 47 points. The higher scores represented institutionally-oriented practices; the lower scores child-centred practices. The possible range was from 0 to 60 points. The scores for each unit were given in Table 10.1 (p. 130). The mean score for the hostels was 11·0 points (SD 6·7 points); for the voluntary homes the mean score was 27·7 points (DS 13·5), and that for the hospitals 43·0 (SD 4·0).

There was no overlap between the scores obtained in the hostels and those in the hospitals, and the difference in mean scores between hostels and hospitals was highly significant statistically ($t = 8.90$, $p < 0.001$). The lowest scoring voluntary home, with 14 points, came well within the range of hostel scores, whereas the highest scoring voluntary home, with 41 points, came within the range of the hospital scores. The third voluntary home, which scored 28 points on the scale, was intermediate between the range of scores obtained by the hostels and the hospitals.

Clearly, the institutions, all of which accommodated retarded children, differed from each other in the patterns of child management which were practised in them. In particular, it is notable that these differences were most clearly marked between institutions of different types, namely the hospitals and the hostels. The voluntary homes do not constitute a clear type, at least in terms of their patterns of care, sometimes approaching the hostel pattern and sometimes the hospital pattern. A comparison of the child management practices in all the units we have studied—those in the field studies as well as the survey—is instructive, and substantially confirms the evidence reported above.

There were only 15 items in the original Child Management Scale which were also used in the revised scale (see p. 109). Scale scores using only these 15 items were therefore calculated for the 16 units in the survey. This enabled us to compare the child management practices in all units studied in the total research programme. The mean scores obtained by the 96 units on the

TABLE 11.1   *Mean unit scores, standard deviations and range of scores on fifteen-item scale of child management for all institutions: field studies and survey*

|  | Establishments | Number of units | Mean score | SD | Range |
|---|---|---|---|---|---|
| Field studies | Children's homes | 57 | 1·78 | 1·56 | 0–6 |
|  | Mental subnormality wards | 15 | 24·20 | 2·51 | 21–28 |
|  | Paediatric wards | 5 | 19·40 | 1·34 | 18–21 |
|  | Local Authority hostel | 1 | 6·00 |  |  |
|  | Voluntary home | 2 | 12·50 | 2·12 | 11–14 |
| Survey | Hostel units | 8 | 5·88 | 4·26 | 0–11 |
|  | Hospital wards | 5 | 22·60 | 0·89 | 22–24 |
|  | Voluntary homes | 3 | 15·70 | 6·66 | 10–23 |

15-item Child Management Scale are presented in Table 11.1 above, along with the standard deviations, the range of scores and the numbers of units which comprised each type of establishment.

The data in Table 11.1 make it clear that child management practices in the five hospital wards investigated in the survey closely resemble those which characterized the fifteen wards of the mental subnormality hospital investigated in the field study. The scores of the five wards fall within the range of the fifteen wards in the field study and, not surprisingly, there is no significant difference between the mean scores of the two groups ($t=1\cdot38$, $p=$N.S.).

The scores of the wards in the paediatric hospital are lower (with the exception of one ward) than the scores of either of the two sets of subnormality wards ($t=3\cdot92$, $p<0\cdot001$). Quite different from the scores of both those types of hospitals are those which characterize the cottages of the two children's homes, the Local Authority hostel in the field study, and the eight Local Authority hostels in the survey. The mean score of the nine hostel units is significantly higher than that which characterizes the children's homes ($t=5\cdot40$, $p<0\cdot001$). The scores of the units in the hostels are, however, much closer to those in the children's homes than they are to the scores obtained by the wards in the subnormality hospitals or the voluntary homes. The voluntary homes span a greater range of scores than any other type of institution, overlapping with the hostels at one extreme and the subnormality hospitals at the other.

Both the data from the fifteen-item scale and the thirty-item scale indicate that different types of establishment have different types of management practices. The children's homes are the most child-oriented, followed by the subnormality hostels; the subnormality voluntary homes, on average, come next, although they overlap greatly with the institutions on either side; then come the paediatric wards, while the most institutionally-oriented are the subnormality hospitals.

## Hypothesis II

Our second hypothesis (p. 122) stated that differences between units in child management practices would not be related to differences in the handicaps of their residents, except in extreme cases. There are many possible handicaps or disabilities which might be thought to present such problems of management that one pattern of care rather than another becomes inevitable or more likely. At the end of the field studies, we concluded that differences in handicaps could not account for the differences in patterns of care between institutions, and in our survey we found no compelling evidence to refute this hypothesis. However, the possible relationships between characteristics of residents and patterns of care are intricate.

If all the ninety-six units studied are compared on the fifteen-item scale as outlined above, it is clear that the relationship between primary handicaps and patterns of care is much weaker than that between type of institution and pattern of care. All of the units in the children's homes contained children of normal intelligence and without physical handicaps, and they scored within the range of 0 to 6 on the scale. The nine Local Authority hostels studied all cared for severely retarded children, yet five of these (four in the survey and one from the field study) scored within the range of the children's homes. They scored 0, 2, 2, 5 and 6 respectively, while the remaining four hostels scored 7, 10, 10 and 11 points. Even the highest scoring hostel was markedly more child-oriented in its patterns of care than the lowest scoring ward in *any* hospital—paediatric or subnormality. Yet the difference—on any interpretation of the severity of handicaps—between the children in the hostels and the homes was clearly much greater than the difference between the children in the hostels and the hospitals.

It is possible, however, that other characteristics of the children influence the types of management practice which are adopted in the living units. Although the majority of children in the units studied in the survey were ambulant and of school age, they were very different from those in the children's homes, not merely because they were retarded, but also because they presented—to a much greater degree—other social and physical problems which had to be dealt with by the staff.

By looking solely at the units in our survey, in which all the children were retarded, we can examine the extent to which the degree of retardation, and other social and physical handicaps, influenced the management practices in the units. In spite of the difficulties experienced in matching units, there were still a number of units in which comparable proportions of children, with specific handicapping conditions, were accommodated. These units differed remarkably in their child management practices, and in the comparisons which follow scores on the thirty-item revised Child Management Scale are used.*

In four units, two hospital wards, one voluntary home and one hostel, the children were similar in terms of their ability to walk unaided and their grade of defect. They differed somewhat in age, ward E containing more older children. There were very big

---

* All further references to the Child Management Scale are to the revised version unless otherwise stated.

141

differences in the child management practices between these units, as reflected in their scale scores. The data are presented in Table 11.2.

TABLE 11.2 *Characteristics of children in four units*

|  |  | Hostel 3 | Vol. home X | Ward D | Ward E |
|---|---|---|---|---|---|
| No. of children |  | 21 | 12 | 26 | 47 |
| Scale scores |  | 14 | 14 | 45 | 41 |
| *Children's characteristics* |  |  |  |  |  |
| Age in years: | 2–4 | 2 | 1 | 2 | 0 |
|  | 5–10 | 16 | 8 | 22 | 12 |
|  | 11–14 | 3 | 3 | 2 | 13 |
|  | 15+ | 0 | 0 | 0 | 22 |
| IQs: | 0–20 | 3 | 2 | 6 | 3 |
|  | 21–30 | 3 | 3 | 6 | 7 |
|  | 31–40 | 6 | 2 | 7 | 18 |
|  | 41–50 | 5 | 3 | 6 | 7 |
|  | 51+ | 1 | 1 | 0 | 1 |
|  | No. info. | 3 | 1 | 1 | 11 |
| Non-ambulant |  | 0 | 2 | 2 | 0 |

The children in the hostel and the voluntary home unit were very similar indeed to those in ward D, although they were perhaps less handicapped than those in ward E. Yet both the hostel and the home had scale scores of 14, as opposed to 45 for ward D. Furthermore, although ward D contained a younger and less difficult-to-manage group of children than ward E, it was actually more institutionally-oriented in its management practices.

If degree of mental defect, ability to walk and age do not seem to influence the child management practices in these units, it is possible to argue that other matters, such as incontinence and behaviour disorders, which present very real problems of management for the staff, would do so. At first sight, our data seemed to give some support to this contention. There were marked differences in the proportions of children in the three types of unit who were incontinent and manifested behaviour disorders, as shown in Table 11.3. Following the definitions employed by Kushlick (1965), incontinence here means that the children were either wet or soiled themselves at least once a week.* Children with behaviour dis-

---

* The data on incontinence were analysed in this way for comparison with Kushlick's data for the Wessex region. It is interesting to note, however, that of the 156 children who were incontinent 'weekly', only 30 of these were incontinent less frequently than once per day.

TABLE 11·3 *Percentages of incontinent and behaviour-disordered children in sixteen institutions*[a]

| | | Incontinent only[b] | Behaviour-disordered only[c] | Incont. & behaviour-dis'd | Total incont. | Total beh.-dis. | Revised C.M.S. scores |
|---|---|---|---|---|---|---|---|
| Hostels | 1 | 13 | 26 | 13 | 26 | 39 | 10 |
| | 2 | 12 | 15 | 0 | 12 | 15 | 6 |
| | 3 | 29 | 10 | 5 | 33 | 14 | 14 |
| | 4 | 0 | 0 | 0 | 0 | 0 | 4 |
| | 5 | 11 | 21 | 11 | 21 | 32 | 22 |
| | 6 | 33 | 13 | 7 | 40 | 20 | 3 |
| | 7 | 0 | 8 | 0 | 0 | 8 | 18 |
| | 8 | 9 | 17 | 4 | 13 | 22 | 11 |
| Mean | | 14·2 | 15·4 | 4·9 | 19·1 | 20·4 | 11·0 |
| Hospitals | A | 31 | 3 | 6 | 38 | 9 | 47 |
| | B | 25 | 11 | 11 | 36 | 23 | 37 |
| | C | 20 | 17 | 44 | 64 | 61 | 45 |
| | D | 62 | 12 | 4 | 66 | 15 | 45 |
| | E | 36 | 17 | 32 | 68 | 49 | 41 |
| Mean | | 32·6 | 12·6 | 22·1 | 54·7 | 34·7 | 43·0 |
| Voluntary homes | X | 25 | 17 | 8 | 33 | 25 | 14 |
| | Y | 95 | 0 | 6 | 100 | 6 | 41 |
| | Z | 80 | 0 | 20 | 100 | 20 | 28 |
| Mean | | 70·0 | 5·0 | 10·0 | 80·0 | 15·0 | 27·7 |

[a] Percentages rounded to nearest whole number.
[b] Incontinence means wetting or soiling at least once per week.
[c] Behaviour disorders means children who exhibit to a marked degree, at least, two of the following: aggression, destructiveness, over-activity, attention-seeking and self-mutilation.

orders were those who exhibited, to a marked degree, at least two of the following problems: aggression, destructiveness, over-activity, attention-seeking behaviour, and self-mutilation.

As the data in Table 11.3 indicate, there was a higher proportion of children in both the hospital wards and the voluntary homes who were incontinent than there was in the hostels. These differences in the prevalence of incontinence between the hospitals and voluntary homes on the one hand and the hostels on the other is statistically significant ($p < 0.001$). When we looked at incontinence in different units in more detail, however, the relationship between incontinence, type of institution and scale score was not so clear-cut. Voluntary home X, hostel 3, and wards A and B all had a third of their children who were wet at least once per week, but they differed markedly in their Child Management Scale scores: both the hostel and the home scored 14 points on the scale, while the two wards scored 47 and 37 points respectively.

As can be seen from Table 11.3, two wards had very high proportions of children with severe behaviour disorders (61 per cent of the children in ward C and 49 per cent of those in ward E). There were no hostel units with as high a proportion of children with behaviour disorders as those wards. Four hostels, however, (1 with 39 per cent, 5 with 32 per cent, 6 with 20 per cent and 8 with 22 per cent), had as high or higher proportions of behaviour-disordered children as the remaining three wards (A with 9 per cent, B with 23 per cent and D with 15 per cent). All of the hostels, nonetheless, had revised Child Management Scale scores lower than any of the wards. Moreover, it is apparent that within institutional types, the scale scores for the units are not related to differences in the proportions of behaviour-disordered children in those units.

We then looked at the possibility that some combination of handicap was associated with patterns of care. When units were compared on the proportions of children who were both incontinent and behaviour disordered, several were found to be similar in this respect. Hospital ward D, for example, had 4 per cent who were both incontinent and behaviour disordered, and so did hostel 8. Yet the revised Child Management Scale scores were 45 in the first case and 11 in the second. Hospital ward B was similar to hostel 5, both with 11 per cent of their children who were incontinent and behaviour disordered. The ward had a scale score of 37 points, while the hostel had a score of 22 points. Again, hospital ward A and hostel 6 were almost identical in the proportions of children they accommodated who were handicapped in this way, with 6 and 7 per cent respectively. The ward scored 47 points on the scale, while the hostel scored 3 points.

Two hospital wards, however, C and E, had considerably more

children in this category than did any other units, having 44 per cent and 32 per cent who were incontinent and behaviour disordered, and they scored 45 points and 41 points on the revised Child Management Scale. It could be argued, therefore, that where the concentration of incontinent and behaviour-disordered children in a unit is as great as this, it is difficult to adopt management practices that are anything but institutionally-oriented. It may be that where a heavy concentration of management problems exists, a much higher staffing ratio is required to maintain a child-oriented pattern of care, but whatever the staffing situation, the converse of this proposition is certainly not true. Units with only very small proportions of children having these disabilities were found which had very institutionally-oriented management patterns. Indeed, it would seem—from the evidence collected in this survey—that child management practices are only weakly related to the handicaps of the residents, and much more strongly related to the type of institution in which they are found.

## Hypothesis III

In our third hypothesis (p. 122), we stated that differences in the child management practices between living units will not be related to the overall size of the establishments of which they are a part.

Size has been measured by the total number of beds available in each institution, regardless of whether they were filled or not at the time of our research. Institutional size was then correlated with scores of the sixteen units on the Child Management Scale. At first sight, it is apparent that the Child Management Scale scores are related to the overall size of the institutions. Figure 11.1 portrays the data.

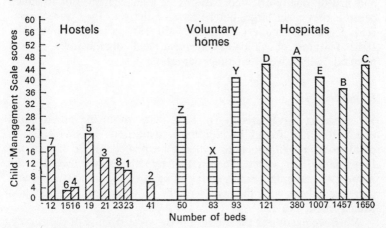

Fig. 11.1 *Scores by institution size*

The rank order correlation between size of institution and scale scores is 0·76, which is significant at the 1 per cent level.

However, if we examine scale scores and institutional size within types of establishments, this relationship no longer holds. If anything, there is a slight tendency for the larger establishments to show greater child orientation in their management patterns. The hostels vary in size from 12 to 41 patients, and have a range of scores from 3 to 22 (r = −0·05, p = N.S.). The hospitals range in size from 121 to 1,650 patients, yet vary in scores only between 37 and 47 points (r = −0·375, p = N.S.). Within the range 12 to 41 and 121 to 1,650, size has no systematic effects on scale scores. There is, of course, no overlap between types of institution either in scores or overall size, and it may be that somewhere between 40 and 120 there is a critical point at which what might be called a qualitative change in child management practices in the living units occurs. The results for the voluntary homes, which were of inter-mediate size, do not suggest that this is the case. Nor do the data from the large children's homes in the field studies support such an hypothesis: each of these had more than 300 children in residence, yet their child management practices were very child-orientated, as we have shown. If we compare the scores those in-stitutions obtained on the fifteen-item scale with those which the five hospitals obtained on the same measure, we find that although there is an overlap in size, both the children's homes being bigger than one of the hospitals, there is no overlap in scores on the Child Management Scale (t = 28·97, p < 0·001).

There are many arguments for and against institutions of different sizes, but we found no systematic relationship between size and child management practices. The large hospitals we studied had institutionally-oriented patterns of management, not so much because they were large, but because of the way they were organized. Even the smallest of them, with 121 patients, showed the same features of child management and organization as the hospitals which were ten times larger.

## Hypothesis IV

We stated in hypothesis IV (p. 122), that, within the broad limits expected to be found in children's institutions in this country, child management practices will not be related to the size of the living units themselves. To test this hypothesis, we recorded the number of patients actually living in each of the units studied and correlated these with the scores of the units on the revised Child Management Scale.

When we examined these data for the sixteen units in the survey, we found that there was a rank order correlation between child management scores and size of units which was significant at the 5-per-cent level ($r=0.45$). However, when we again looked at this more closely within types of institutions, the relationship between scale scores and unit size disappears. Again within intitutional type, there is a tendency for child management practices to become more child-oriented as unit size increases, though this was not statistically significant. This can be clearly seen in Fig. 11.2 below, from which the voluntary homes have been omitted.

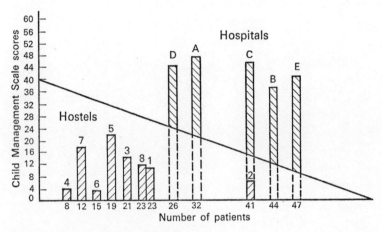

Fig. 11.2 *Scores by size of living units*

The hostels, in the lower diagonal of Fig. 11.2, vary in unit size from 8 to 41 patients but none scores higher on the scale than 22 points ($r=0.04$, $p=$N.S.) The hospitals, in the upper diagonal, range in size of wards from 26 to 47 patients, but none scores less than 37 points on the scale ($r=-0.68$, $p=$N.S.). There is a clear overlap in unit size between the two types of institution, but the patterns of scale scores are markedly different. The voluntary homes have not been included in the diagram for the sake of simplicity, but there was also no systematic relationship between size of units and scale scores for these institutions.

The apparent association between scale scores and unit size, therefore, appears to be a by-product of the association between scale scores and institutional type, in much the same way as we found for the association between scale scores and overall size.

Once again, there are many other arguments for and against

147

units of different sizes, and the fact that we could find no systematic relationship between size and scale scores does not mean that the size of unit is of no importance. We return to this matter in our concluding chapter.

# 12   Staffing and child management

Mental subnormality hospitals are chronically short of staff, particularly nurses. As was noted in Chapter 6, for example, over the period January to March 1964, the nursing staff in the combined hospital was 14·2 per cent below establishment. (By 1966, the average figure for the same three months was only 3·7 per cent below establishment, but the point still holds.) Recent surveys all emphasize the importance of shortage of staff and its relation to poor child management practices—see Martin, Bone and Spain (1971), Morris (1969), Ely Hospital Inquiry (1969). The way in which staff are able to look after children must obviously be influenced by the numbers of children each staff member has to cope with. However, in dealing with young or handicapped children, a high staff-child ratio may be a necessary but not a sufficient condition for child-oriented management.

The children's wards which we studied were comparatively well staffed by British standards: and indeed, in British hospitals for the mentally retarded one does not find in the children's wards the same very great shortage of nursing staff which is so character-istic a feature of many North American and some European institutions (Wolfensberger, 1969), though our staffing ratios compare unfavourably with those found in other European coun-tries (Nirje, 1969). How were the hospitals and hostels which we studied in our survey staffed, and were there differences between them which could account for differences in child management?

We put forward three hypotheses (V, VI and VII in Chapter 9) concerned with staff numbers and their deployment. The first was that there would be no difference in the *assigned* staff-child ratios between institutions with child-oriented, and those with institution-ally-oriented, child management practices. The second was that the

149

*effective* staff ratios would differ—that is, the numbers of staff on duty at different times of the day would be different in the two types of institution. Specifically, it was predicted that units characterized by child-oriented practices would have most staff on duty during peak periods (that is, periods in which there were most children about, and when the child-care activities demanded a high staff ratio if children were to get individual attention). The third hypothesis was that there would be greater continuity of staff in units characterized by child-oriented management practices.

## Hypothesis V

We calculated *assigned* staff-child ratios, excluding domestic helpers and night staff, for the week in each institution in which the field-work took place. *Assigned* staff ratios, as discussed in Chapter 6, take account only of staff actually allocated to work in the units, so that the measure used here was not the simple count of total staff divided by patients, which has been used by some investigators, for example Ullmann (1967). For each unit, we worked out the number of 'full-time equivalent' staff as follows. Each person who worked 40 or more hours on the ward during that week was counted as one full-time staff member. Those working between 30 and 39 hours counted as 0·8; 20–29 hours as 0·6; 10–19 as 0·4; and less than 10 hours as 0·2 staff members. Because in some units the children went home at weekends, only weekdays were included in this analysis. The results are presented in Table 12.1.

For the hospitals, the average number of children per staff member, as calculated above, ranged from 3·42 to 8·15, mean 5·36. For the hostels, the range was 2·50, to 8·91, mean 5·11. For the three voluntary homes, the range was 3·17 to 9·00, mean 5·34. The hostels had a better staff ratio than hospitals, but none of the differences between the three types of institutions was statistically significant.* Within types of institution, there was even a slight but not significant tendency for units in which each staff member had, on average, a *larger* number of children to care

* It was pointed out to us (by Dr Albert Kushlick), after these data were first published (King and Raynes, 1968c), that by taking 40 hours or more per week as the Full Time Equivalent, we might be underestimating the staff ratios in the hostels, where staff worked longer hours. We therefore re-calculated F.T.E. as follows: where staff worked 40–49 hours, this was counted as 1·0; 50–59 as 1·2 and 60–69 as 1·4 staff, to eliminate any possibility of bias. This did indeed affect the ratios in three hostels, but only marginally, and this in no way affected any statistical calculations: unit 4 had a ratio of 1:2·67 on this basis (instead of 1:2·86), unit 6 had a ratio of 1:4·69 (instead of 1:5·36) and unit 7 a ratio of 1:4·29 (instead of 1:4·62). The mean ratio for the hostels thus became 1:4·96. Although it is true that the hostel staff work longer hours per week, this factor had already been largely eliminated by confining the comparison to weekdays.

for to be characterized by *more* child-oriented practices: the correlation with hospitals between revised Child Management Scales scores and child-staff ratios was r= −0·63 and that between hostels was r= −0·31. Neither of these correlations was statistically significant, and it may be concluded that within the limits of staffing explored in this enquiry, there was no relation between *assigned* child-staff ratios and child management practices.

TABLE 12.1 *Assigned staff to child ratios (weekdays) in sixteen institutions*

|  |  | No. of assigned F.T.E. staff[a] | No. of children | Ratio children to 1 staff |
|---|---|---|---|---|
| Hostels | 1 | 3·4 | 23 | 6·76 |
|  | 2 | 4·6 | 41 | 8·91 |
|  | 3 | 8·4 | 21 | 2·50 |
|  | 4 | 2·8 | 8 | 2·86 |
|  | 5 | 4·6 | 19 | 4·13 |
|  | 6 | 2·8 | 15 | 5·36 |
|  | 7 | 2·6 | 12 | 4·62 |
|  | 8 | 4·0 | 23 | 5·75 |
| Totals |  | 33·2 | 162 | 40·89 |
| Means |  | 4·15 | 20·25 | 5·11 |
| Hospitals | A | 6·2 | 32 | 5·16 |
|  | B | 5·4 | 44 | 8·15 |
|  | C | 10·6 | 41 | 3·87 |
|  | D | 7·6 | 26 | 3·42 |
|  | E | 7·6 | 47 | 6·18 |
| Totals |  | 37·4 | 190 | 26·78 |
| Means |  | 7·48 | 38 | 5·36 |
| Voluntary homes | X | 3·8 | 12 | 3·17 |
|  | Y | 2·0 | 18 | 9·00 |
|  | Z | 2·6 | 10 | 3·85 |
| Totals |  | 8·4 | 40 | 16·02 |
| Means |  | 2·8 | 13·3 | 5·34 |

[a]F.T.E. equivalents were calculated as follows: less than 10 hours = 0·2 staff; 1–19 hours = 0·4; 20–29 = 0·6: 30–39 = 0·8; and 40 or more hours = 1·0 staff.

## Hypothesis VI

*Assigned* staff child ratios in themselves tell us how many children have to be looked after by the equivalent of one full-time member

151

of staff during the course of one week. In practice, however, available staff were used somewhat differently so that the staffing complement within a unit differed markedly at different times of the day in most units.

We made a systematic study of this matter. Form C1 (p. 221) provided a staff timetable for each day, divided into half-hour periods for each unit. On this form, we recorded which members of staff were on duty for all the half-hourly intervals during the week of the fieldwork. Information was obtained from the head of the unit about the number of children present in the unit at different periods of the day, and the timing of specific activities was obtained by interview and by observation. As a result, our data made it possible to relate the number of staff on duty to the numbers of children and the activities going on in the unit at those times, in the form of *effective* staff ratios.*

In the event, we decided to examine two 'peak' periods, when all the children would be present and the units were at their busiest, and two 'slack' periods, when those children who went to school or training centres were away from their units, leaving fewer children to be cared for. The 'peak' periods were from 7.30 a.m. to 9.30 a.m., and from 4.30 p.m. to 6.30 p.m. Although there were some differences in the routines from unit to unit, the morning peak period involved getting the children up, washing and breakfast and getting those children who went to school ready to leave the unit. The evening peak period, in most units, included such activities as giving the children tea, washing or bathing the children and getting at least the younger ones ready for bed. All of the children were present in their units during these times. Table 12.2 presents the *effective* staff ratios for all units for both peak periods.†

When the *effective* ratios for morning and evening peak periods are compared with the *assigned* ratios for living units (given in

* Mean numbers of staff were calculated for each interval over the five days of the fieldwork. In four hostels, where there were no children present on Monday mornings and Friday afternoons because the children went home for weekends, the calculation was made over a four-day period.

† We also calculated effective staff ratios for peak and slack periods, using the activities being carried out as the basis for comparison, rather than strictly similar time intervals. Thus, we calculated how many staff hours per child were involved in one unit which took two hours to get the children up, and compared that with the staff hours per child in another unit, which completed the same process in, say, one and a quarter hours, and so on. Very similar results were achieved in that way – see Raynes (1968). Since the time intervals used in the present discussion cover closely similar areas of activity in all units, the simpler technique of comparing the same time intervals has been preferred here. It enables us to use the more readily understandable concept of numbers of children per member of staff instead of numbers of staff hours per child.

| | No. children in unit | a.m. peak[a] | | p.m. peak[a] | |
| --- | --- | --- | --- | --- | --- |
| | | Mean staff on duty | Ratio children to 1 staff | Mean staff on duty | Ratio children to 1 staff |
| Hostels[b] 1 | 23 | 3·00 | 7·67 | 2·80 | 8·21 |
| 2 | 41 | 6·00 | 6·83 | 5·00 | 8·20 |
| 3 | 21 | 6·30 | 3·33 | 4·52 | 4·65 |
| 4 | 8 | 2·20 | 3·63 | 2·16 | 3·70 |
| 5 | 19 | 4·00 | 4·75 | 3·80 | 5·00 |
| 6 | 15 | 2·75 | 5·45 | 2·00 | 7·50 |
| 7 | 12 | 1·75 | 6·86 | 3·00 | 4·00 |
| 8 | 23 | 3·75 | 6·13 | 3·72 | 6·18 |
| Totals | 162 | 29·75 | 44·65 | 27·00 | 47·44 |
| Means | 20·25 | 3·72 | 5·58 | 3·38 | 5·93 |
| Hospitals A | 32 | 3·95 | 8·10 | 2·72 | 11·76 |
| B | 44 | 3·65 | 12·05 | 2·92 | 15·07 |
| C | 41 | 5·40 | 7·59 | 4·52 | 9·07 |
| D | 26 | 6·60 | 3·94 | 3·88 | 6·70 |
| E | 47 | 4·55 | 10·33 | 4·16 | 11·29 |
| Totals | 190 | 24·15 | 42·01 | 18·30 | 53·89 |
| Means | 38 | 4·83 | 8·40 | 3·64 | 10·78 |
| Voluntary homes X | 12 | 2·35 | 5·11 | 2·56 | 4·69 |
| Y | 18 | 1·50 | 12·00 | 1·00 | 18·00 |
| Z | 10 | 2·10 | 4·76 | 1·24 | 8·06 |
| Totals | 40 | 5·95 | 21·87 | 4·80 | 30·75 |
| Means | 13·3 | 1·98 | 7·29 | 1·60 | 10·25 |

[a] A.m. peak period 7.30 a.m. – 9.30 a.m., p.m. peak period 4.30 p.m. – 6.30 p.m.
[b] For 4 hostels, where the children went home at weekends, the mean numbers of staff were calculated over 4 days; in all other units over 5 days of the fieldwork.

153

Table 12.1), it is apparent that, for most units, the *assigned* ratios give a more favourable impression of staffing than is really the case. Nearly all the units are better staffed in the morning period than they are during the evening peak, but there are wide differences between units of different types. The hostels were one-and-a-half times as well staffed as the hospitals during the morning peak period ($t = 2 \cdot 17$, $p < 0 \cdot 1$, $df = 11$), and one-and-three-quarter times as well staffed during the evening peak ($t = 3 \cdot 51$, $p < 0 \cdot 01$, $df = 11$). Although the rank order correlation between *effective* staff ratios for the morning period and revised Child Management Scale scores was in the expected direction, this was not significant statistically. For the evening period, the correlation between staff ratios and scale scores was $r = 0 \cdot 49$, $p < 0 \cdot 05$. There were no significant correlations when we examined scale scores and staff ratios within the hostels as a group and within the hospitals as a group.

The *effective* staff ratios for the peak periods were then compared with the *effective* staff ratios during the two slack periods. The idea was to see whether staffing was reduced during slack periods and increased during peak periods. The 'slack' periods were from 9.30 to 11.30 in the morning and from 1.30 to 3.30 in the afternoons. In the hostels, all of the children were away from the living units at these times: in the hospitals, the numbers on the wards were reduced by between 25 and 80 per cent. One voluntary home had the same number of children on the unit at all times, and the voluntary homes were therefore excluded from this analysis.

During the morning, in both the hospitals and the hostels, there was virtually no difference in the staffing between peak and slack periods. The hostels, on average, had slightly fewer staff on duty during the slack period, $3 \cdot 57$, than during the peak period, $3 \cdot 72$; in the hospitals there were, on average, $4 \cdot 86$ staff during the slack period, as against $4 \cdot 83$ during the peak period. In the afternoons, however, the situation was very different. The mean number of staff on duty in the slack period for the hostels was $2 \cdot 21$ — a reduction of about 35 per cent from the mean number of $3 \cdot 38$ for the peak period. In four out of the five hospital wards, on the other hand, there were actually *fewer* staff on duty during the peak evening period than there had been during the afternoon slack period. The mean number of staff for the hospital slack period was $4 \cdot 91$, and for the peak period only $3 \cdot 64$.

These findings confirm Hypothesis VI, that although there was no differences in the total numbers of full-time equivalent staff *assigned* to the units, the more child-oriented units would have higher *effective* staff ratios at the times they were most needed.

These differences in *effective* staff ratios obviously reflect the different arrangements for the off-duty of full-time staff and the organization of part-time staff in different establishments.

The lower *effective* staff-child ratios for the hospitals during the evenings can be accounted for to a large extent by the working of the 'shift' system, which operated in four of the hospitals we studied. Under the shift system, two sets of staff worked on altern-ate shifts on alternate weeks: one shift worked five mornings (from 7.30 a.m. until 2 p.m.) with one long day (7.30 a.m. until 5.30 p.m. or, in some cases, 6 p.m.) and one day off; the other shift worked five afternoons (from 12.30 p.m. until 8.30 p.m.) with one long day (7.30 a.m. until 5.30 p.m. or 6 p.m.) and one day off. This system meant that, each day, the ward team was depleted by at least one member of staff at the crucial time of 5.30 p.m. or 6 p.m. In the hostels the staff were on duty from the time the children got up until the time they went to bed, with usually two days off (sometimes three and sometimes only one) each week. During the mornings, when the children were at the training centre, hostel staff were engaged in housework and the preparation of the midday meal for the children. In the afternoons, however, they were given time off duty. One hospital operated on a 'long day' system, not unlike the hostels—staff worked from 7.30 a.m. until 8.30 p.m. for three days one week and four days the next. This unit had a much higher number of staff on duty at peak periods than the other four hospitals, and was, in this respect, comparable to the hostels. That it did not enjoy a child-oriented pattern of care, in spite of high effective staffing, suggests that other factors are more important in explaining patterns of care.

Although long-day systems lend themselves more easily to child-oriented management practices than do shift systems, it must be said that the long day itself is a great strain, and that staff may well find the arrangements for off-duty periods inconvenient. The organization of staff is undoubtedly a difficult problem in which the interests of the children have to be balanced against the needs of the staff. It may be that a greater use of part-time staff at peak periods is required to make up any deficiencies.

*Hypothesis VII*

According to this hypothesis (p. 122), we expected to find greater continuity of staff in child-oriented units than in institutionally-oriented units, and it was the case that the staffing of hostels was much more stable than that for hospitals.

An indication of the extreme instability of staffing in some units can be gained by simply counting the numbers of different

155

staff members employed in different units during the week in which the fieldwork took place. The figures are given in Table 12.3 for each unit. The table excludes domestics and night staff.

TABLE 12.3  *Numbers of staff employed in units during week of fieldwork*

| Hostels | | | Hospitals | | | Voluntary homes | | |
|---|---|---|---|---|---|---|---|---|
| Unit | staff | children | Unit | staff | children | Unit | staff | children |
| 1 | 8 | 23 | A | 12 | 32 | X | 4 | 12 |
| 2 | 6 | 41 | B | 9 | 44 | Y | 5 | 18 |
| 3 | 14 | 21 | C | 29[a] | 41 | Z | 7 | 10 |
| 4 | 3 | 8 | D | 13 | 26 | | | |
| 5 | 5 | 19 | E | 15 | 47 | | | |
| 6 | 3 | 15 | | | | | | |
| 7 | 4 | 12 | | | | | | |
| 8 | 7 | 23 | | | | | | |
| Total 8 | 50 | 162 | 5 | 88 | 190 | 3 | 16 | 40 |
| Means 1 | 6·25 | 20·25 | 1 | 17·6 | 38·0 | 1 | 5·3 | 13·3 |

[a]It seems likely that the numbers of staff in this unit were exceptionally high during the week of the fieldwork.

The table shows that in one week, children in the hospitals have dealings with much larger numbers of staff (on average 17·6) than do children in the hostels (on average 6·25) or voluntary homes (5·3). These differences in part reflect differences in the size of living units, but there are some marked inconsistencies. Thus, hostel 2 has forty-one children, but only six different staff were on duty during the week, whereas hospital C, in what was surely an exceptional week, had no fewer than twenty-nine different staff on duty for forty-one children. Hostel 8, with twenty-three children, had seven staff, whereas hospital B, with twenty-six children, had thirteen. All of the hostels except one had smaller numbers of different staff on duty during the week than any of the hospitals.

We made another estimate of staff continuity by calculating an 'expected' number of staff who would work in a unit during a period of six months. This was done by asking heads of units to give us the names of all staff who had joined the unit after the fieldwork period, and who had either left or who were still there in the week ending 16 September 1967. As the number of weeks comprising this period was known, it was possible to estimate an expected number of new staff in a period of 26 weeks. There were some variations in the number of weeks for which data were provided, the range being 16–26 weeks, and this could, of course, affect the numbers of new staff reported. The estimates are given in Table 12.4. Although these estimates must be regarded as subject to some error, they do show a striking difference between the hospitals and the hostels.

TABLE 12.4    *Estimated numbers of new staff expected in a six-month period for all sixteen institutions*[a]

| | Hostels | | Hospitals | | Voluntary homes | |
| | | Expected | | Expected | | Expected |
| Unit | new staff | Unit | new staff | Unit | new staff |
|---|---|---|---|---|---|
| 1 | 1·0 | A | 7·0 | X | 7·8 |
| 2 | 4·7 | B | 39·5 | Y | 1·0 |
| 3 | 3·9 | C | 19·2 | Z | 1·6 |
| 4 | 0·0 | D | 8·1 | | |
| 5 | 0·0 | E | 29·1 | | |
| 6 | 0·0 | | | | |
| 7 | 0·0 | | | | |
| 8 | 2·9 | | | | |
| Totals   8 | 12·5 | 5 | 102·9 | 3 | 10·4 |
| Means   1 | 1·6 | 1 | 20·6 | 1 | 3·5 |

[a]Estimates are based on new staff joining in period ranging from 16–26 weeks after fieldwork completed.

As a group, the hospitals wards are likely to have thirteen times as many new staff working in them over a 6-month period as the hostels and six times as many as the voluntary homes. Continuity in child care is clearly more likely to be found in the hostels and the voluntary homes than it is in the hospitals, where children are likely to be cared for by, on average, more than twenty new members of staff during a period of 6 months. If we add to these night staff—who have an important role to play in the lives of the children—and domestics, it is possible that, in some hospitals for the retarded, the children may have to adjust to as many as a hundred different adults during the course of a year.

# 13 Staff roles and the way they are performed

The analysis so far has shown that differences in the patterns of care between hospitals, hostels and voluntary homes cannot be explained simply in terms of the size of the institutions, the size of the living units or the numbers available to staff them. Each of these factors, in their different ways, may have important implications for the long-term care of children, though none of them provides an adequate explanation for the differences in practices as measured by the revised Child Management Scale. Some evidence was reported in the last chapter, however, which suggests that the way in which the available staff are deployed in each unit is related to the pattern of care which prevails. We now turn to an examination of what the staff actually do within the units and how they carry out their tasks, in relation to the patterns of care.

At the end of the field studies, we had formed the impression that child-oriented units showed many features of what we called 'household organization', whereas institutionally-oriented units did not. In the former, all grades of staff seemed to participate in most activities of the unit, and the heads of units were closely involved in the everyday care of the children, in addition to their administrative, budgetary and other responsibilities. In the latter, there appeared to be a marked division of labour between different grades of staff, and heads of units seemed to be only marginally involved in the everyday care of children. We formulated these impressions more precisely as Hypotheses VIII, IX, X and XI in Chapter 9, and the evidence in relation to these hypotheses is reviewed here.

## Collecting the data

Our data in relation to staff activities were collected from systematic observations carried out over two mornings and two afternoons in each living unit. The method of observing was outlined in Chapter 10. In brief, staff were divided into three status groups: head of unit, junior child care staff and domestic staff, and a representative from each group was observed, in rotation, so that a third of our observations related to each group. Observation intervals lasted for 30 seconds, followed by 30 seconds for recording, and three consecutive observations were made of the activities of one person before attention was shifted to another staff member in a different status group. During the mornings, the observations began at the time the children got up, and continued until they went to school, or until 10.30 a.m. in cases where there were no schoolchildren; in the afternoons, they started when the children returned from school (or 4 p.m.) and continued until the last child went to bed (or until 8 p.m., whichever was the earlier). An additional observation period of one hour in the morning and one hour in the afternoon was carried out in the units where there were children who did not go to school. Activities were classified in five categories: Social Child Care; Physical Child Care; Supervision of Children; Domestic Activity and Administration. Each category was denotatively defined by a check list of activities. An additional category, which was not used in the analysis, but which we found necessary for data collection purposes, was labelled 'miscellaneous' and included chit-chat between staff when they were not doing anything else, staff tea breaks, staff talking to the observers, and so on.

A note was made of whether children were present during all activities, and, if so, whether any interaction between staff and children took place. If, during a 30-second period, a member of staff spoke to a child, this fact was also recorded. We made no attempt to document what was said, but we did rate the quality of interaction, whether verbal or physical, within each interval as *rejecting, tolerating* or *accepting*. A complete set of instructions for the conduct of the observations is reproduced in Appendix III (pp. 233–44).

## The analysis

The number of observation periods differed in different wards, because the children got up, went to school, returned from school and went to bed at different times. Although the *functional* periods were the same, the time periods were not identical. Results were therefore expressed in percentage terms as follows: the number of occasions on which an activity *was* observed was divided by the total number of observation intervals during which it *could* have occurred for each category of staff, and this proportion was expressed as a percentage. It sometimes happened that a member of staff was involved in more than one activity during a 30-second observation period—for example, she might start by preparing a meal (Domestic) and then go on to show a child how it is done (Social Child Care). This happened more frequently in the hostels than in the hospitals, but even in the hostels it occurred in only about 12 per cent of the observational periods. As we had no basis for assigning priority to one type of activity rather than another, both types were recorded and counted for those periods. In consequence percentages do not add up to 100. This is not an objection to the method of analysis, which was concerned with the number of *occasions* during which an activity occurred, rather than with the length of *time* that it lasted. Nonetheless, for all practical purposes the proportion of total observation intervals in which each activity was recorded may be taken as closely approximating the proportion of time spent on each type of task, and for convenience we refer to it as such.

A more difficult problem arose in attempting to categorize activities which would more realistically be described as 'doing nothing'. However, on most of these occasions the staff member was nominally doing something (usually supervising children), and was credited accordingly. In practice the procedures used were found to be highly reliable, and even where the subjective rating of the quality of interaction was called for, there was a very high measure of agreement between observers. A full discussion of the reliability of the observations, including the reliability co-efficient for each type, appears in Appendix III.

In the event, insufficient observations of domestic staff were obtained for some units (because of their duty hours), and domestic staff have therefore been excluded from the comparative analysis. To simplify the presentation of results most comparisons will be confined to the hostels and hospitals. The three voluntary homes were too few in number, and too heterogeneous in structure and organization, to constitute a meaningful group, and the information collected from them can best be used for illustrative purposes (although voluntary home X might well have been included in the analysis with the hostels, since it closely resembled them in many respects).

It is important to note that although we observed individual members of staff to collect our data, we were interested not in the members of staff themselves but in the *roles* which they were required to perform and which they had been trained to carry out. It follows that our findings reflect not on the kindliness or dedication of individuals, but on the operational structures within which they were required to work, and the training programmes which were designed to support them. Obviously, individuals were able to influence these structures to some extent, but our data show, for the most part, that individual differences were greatly outweighed by structural constraints.

*Hypothesis VIII*

According to this hypothesis (see p. 123) we expected the role activities of senior staff to be related to the patterns of management in the following way. In units with child-oriented patterns of care, we predicted, the head of the unit will spend a higher proportion of her activities involved in social and physical care and supervision of the children than the heads of institutionally-oriented units. The latter will spend a greater proportion of their activities on administrative or domestic duties, which will not bring them into direct contact with the children.

In order to test this hypothesis, we first calculated the proportion of her time which the head of each unit spent in Social and Physical Child Care, Supervision of Children, Domestic and Administrative duties.* Table 13.1 gives the activities for unit heads in all sixteen units together with the revised Child Management Scale scores.

Correlation coefficients were calculated for each of the head of unit activities and scale scores. Rank order correlations (Spearman) are quoted here, although similar results were found with product moment correlations (Pearson)—indeed, the latter were slightly more significant statistically. We found that the higher the proportion of time the head of the unit spent in Social Child Care and Supervision of Children, the lower (more child-oriented) were the scores of those units on the revised Child Management Scale. For Social Child Care, the correlation was 0·51, and for Supervision 0·49, both of which were significant at the 5 per cent level. On the other hand, the proportion of time spent in Administration was negatively correlated with scores on the scale ($r = -0·53$, $p < 0·05$). Physical Child Care activities and Domestic duties were not, by themselves, related to scale scores. When we combined activities which necessarily involved the head of the unit with children,

---

* Strictly speaking, as noted above, it is the proportion of total observation intervals in which these activities were recorded rather than proportions of total time. We refer to 'time' here and elsewhere simply for the sake of convenient expression. For all practical purposes they are equivalent.

TABLE 13.1   Activities of head of unit and revised Child Management Scale scores in sixteen institutions[a]

| Type of establishment | Rev. C.M.S. scores | Social Child Care | Physical Child Care | Supervisory Child Care | Domestic Activity | Administrative Activity | Social+Physical +Supervisory | Domestic+ Administrative |
|---|---|---|---|---|---|---|---|---|
| Hostels 1 | 10 | 33 | 33 | 25 | 13 | 4 | 90 | 17 |
| 2 | 6 | 8 | 22 | 12 | 39 | 26 | 42 | 65 |
| 3 | 14 | 35 | 22 | 40 | 13 | 17 | 96 | 29 |
| 4 | 4 | 24 | 23 | 24 | 28 | 9 | 72 | 37 |
| 5 | 22 | 22 | 20 | 29 | 14 | 18 | 71 | 32 |
| 6 | 3 | 11 | 31 | 34 | 41 | 7 | 75 | 48 |
| 7 | 18 | 31 | 13 | 34 | 21 | 3 | 78 | 24 |
| 8 | 11 | 21 | 19 | 51 | 13 | 19 | 90 | 32 |
| Hospitals A | 47 | 0 | 33 | 10 | 35 | 27 | 43 | 62 |
| B | 37 | 27 | 14 | 25 | 21 | 25 | 65 | 46 |
| C | 45 | 4 | 14 | 14 | 33 | 44 | 32 | 76 |
| D | 45 | 13 | 5 | 13 | 20 | 51 | 31 | 72 |
| E | 41 | 1 | 9 | 21 | 15 | 43 | 31 | 58 |
| Voluntary X | 14 | 17 | 33 | 16 | 32 | 8 | 67 | 40 |
| homes Y | 41 | 2 | 65 | 2 | 28 | 5 | 69 | 33 |
| Z | 28 | 10 | 36 | 27 | 39 | 9 | 73 | 48 |

[a]Figures have been rounded to nearest whole number. Rows do not add up to 100 because more than one activity could occur in each time interval (see text).

162

and compared them with those that need not involve the children, substantial support was found for the hypothesis. The greater the time spent in Social and Physical Child Care and Supervision by unit heads, the more child-oriented were their units ($r = 0.59$, $p < 0.05$) while the greater the time the unit heads spent on Administrative or Domestic duties, the more institutionally-oriented were their units ($r = -0.45$, $p < 0.05$).

We then compared hostels as a group on the one hand with hospitals as a group on the other. The data are presented in Table 13.2. There were statistically significant differences between the two types of institution in the amount of time spent on Social Child Care and Supervision of Children, heads of units in hostels spending, on average, twice as much of their time on each of these activities as did sisters and charge nurses in hospitals. Heads of hostel units did one-and-a half times as much Physical Child Care as did the heads of hospital units. In both types of unit, senior staff spent about the same amount of time on Domestic Activities—this occured during one-quarter of all observation periods. More than a third of the observed activities of ward sisters were Administrative, and they were three times as likely to be doing work of this kind as were senior staff in the hostels. This difference was highly significant statistically. When we combined activities in the same way as before, and compared them in hostels and hospitals, very clear differences were found.

TABLE 13.2 *Activities of head of unit: hostels and hospitals*[a]

| Activity | 1 Hostels | | 2 Hospitals | | Differences 1–2 | $t$ | $p <$ |
|---|---|---|---|---|---|---|---|
| | $\bar{x}$ | SD | $\bar{x}$ | SD | | | |
| Social Child Care | 23 | 10 | 9 | 11 | +14 | 2·35 | 0·05 |
| Physical Child Care | 23 | 6 | 15 | 11 | +8 | 1·69 | NS |
| Supervisory Child Care | 31 | 12 | 16 | 6 | +15 | 2·53 | 0·05 |
| Domestic Duties | 23 | 12 | 25 | 9 | −2 | 0·37 | NS |
| Administration | 13 | 8 | 38 | 11 | −25 | 4·59 | 0·001 |
| Social + Physical + Supervisory | 77 | 17 | 40 | 15 | +37 | 3·61 | 0·01 |
| Domestic + Administrative | 36 | 15 | 63 | 12 | −27 | 3·18 | 0·01 |

[a]Means ($\bar{x}$). standard deviations (SD) and differences have been rounded to nearest whole number. Columns do not add to 100 because more than one activity could occur in each time interval (see text). Degrees of freedom = 11.

Heads of hostels were engaged in Social, Physical and Supervisory child care in 77 per cent of their observation periods, compared to 40 per cent of the observations for head of wards (t=3·61, p<0·01, df=11): hostel heads were engaged in Domestic or Administrative activity for 36 per cent of the time, compared to 63 per cent for heads of wards (t=3·18, p<0·01, df=11).

Finally, we looked at the hostels and the hospitals separately to see if the relationship between activities of the head of the unit and patterns of management held good within institutional types. The numbers were, of course, very small, and although most of the correlations were in the expected directions, none reached statistical significance.

## Hypothesis IX

According to Hypothesis IX (p. 123), we expected to find differences between institutionally-oriented and child-oriented units in the way the respective unit heads actually carried out their activities. The way staff carry out their activities we have termed *role performance*. We predicted that the heads of child-oriented units, whatever the nature of their activities, would spend a greater part of their time in the presence of children than the heads of institutionally-oriented units. Moreover, when they were with them, their interaction was expected to be characterized by more warmth and a greater frequency of talk than would be the case for the heads of institutionally-oriented units.

Several indices were used to test this hypothesis. First, we examined the proportion of observation periods when children were seen in the same location as unit heads. Second, we looked at the frequency of talking to the children during the times when children were present. Third, we rated the quality of interaction between staff and children whenever it occurred; and lastly, we looked in more detail at those activities which did not *necessarily* involve children (i.e. Domestic and Administrative duties) to see whether they were carried out in such a way that the children were involved, or whether children were excluded from them entirely. The data for each of these indices are given in Table 13.3.

The same kinds of analysis were carried out with these data as those discussed in relation to Hypothesis VIII. There was no significant association between the proportion of observation periods when children were seen with the head of the unit and scores on the revised Child Management Scale, although the correlation was in the expected direction (r=0·38, p=NS). However, the greater frequency of talking to the children during those same

| Type of establishment | 1<br>Rev.<br>C.M.S.<br>scores | 2<br>Children<br>present[b] | 3<br>Staff<br>talked[c] | 4<br>Evaluation[d]<br>Reject | Tolerate | Accept | 5<br>% of Dom. &<br>Admin. activity<br>with interaction[e] |
|---|---|---|---|---|---|---|---|
| Hostels 1 | 10 | 92 | 94 | 6 | 58 | 36 | 42 |
| 2 | 6 | 53 | 88 | 12 | 57 | 31 | 39 |
| 3 | 14 | 86 | 96 | 4 | 52 | 44 | 28 |
| 4 | 4 | 74 | 88 | 11 | 70 | 19 | 57 |
| 5 | 22 | 66 | 83 | 17 | 65 | 17 | 20 |
| 6 | 3 | 81 | 96 | 8 | 36 | 56 | 66 |
| 7 | 18 | 80 | 85 | 15 | 48 | 38 | 35 |
| 8 | 11 | 88 | 94 | 6 | 59 | 35 | 27 |
| Hospitals A | 47 | 69 | 54 | 42 | 55 | 4 | 15 |
| B | 37 | 75 | 83 | 20 | 37 | 44 | 37 |
| C | 45 | 64 | 65 | 31 | 58 | 11 | 33 |
| D | 45 | 47 | 58 | 39 | 42 | 19 | 12 |
| E | 41 | 42 | 61 | 29 | 61 | 11 | 27 |
| Voluntary X | 14 | 76 | 92 | 11 | 71 | 18 | 48 |
| homes Y | 41 | 93 | 32 | 32 | 57 | 11 | 8 |
| | 28 | 87 | 82 | 14 | 73 | 14 | 36 |

[a]Figures have been rounded to nearest whole number.
[b]Column 2 gives the proportion of observation periods in which children were present.
[c]Column 3 expresses the occasions when children were spoken to as a proportion of the occasions when they were present (column 2) and therefore *could* have been spoken to.
[d]The three sets of figures in column 4 give the ratings of interaction when children were present (column 2). The rows here do add up to 100 (apart from rounding) because only one rating per interval was allowed.
[e]Column 5 gives the proportion of Domestic and Administrative activities in which interaction with the children also took place. The base for this calculation is thus the last column in Table 13.1.

165

observation periods was strongly associated with child-oriented practice as measured by the scale ($r = 0.83$, $p < 0.001$).

The quality of any interaction, talk as well as other kinds of contact, was rated for each interval in which it occurred in one of three categories: *rejecting,* which included ignoring the children, failing to respond to their overtures and telling them off; *tolerating,* in which staff initiated purely functional interaction, or responded to the overtures of children with simple acknowledgement; or *accepting,* which involved positive or playful contact between staff and children. (Fuller definitions and the reliability coefficients for these ratings are given in Appendix III.) The proportion of intervals rated as *tolerating* was not associated with scale scores, but both the remaining categories were significantly correlated with scale scores in the predicted directions. The greater the proportion of interactions between unit heads and children which were rated as *accepting,* the more child-oriented were patterns of care ($r = 0.64$, $p < 0.01$); conversely, the greater the proportion of interactions which were rated as *rejecting,* the more institutionally-oriented were patterns of care ($r = -0.85$, $p < 0.001$).

We have already demonstrated, in relation to Hypothesis VIII, that unit heads of institutionally-oriented units spent more time than their counterparts in child oriented units on Domestic and Administrative activities. Since some domestic work and some administration is inevitable in *any* unit, and since these activities could be carried out either with the children or in isolation from them, we decided to look more closely at these activities to see if the way in which unit heads carried them out was different in different types of unit. We found that it was, and that the differences were associated with scores on the revised Child Management Scale. The greater the proportion of the head of the unit's Domestic and Administrative activity which was carried out at the same time as maintaining a contact with the children, the more child-oriented were the patterns of care ($r = 0.76$, $p < 0.01$).

We then compared the role performance of the heads of hostel units with that of the heads of hospital units on each of these four indices. The results are presented in Table 13.4, and require little further discussion. Heads of hostel units spent more of their time with the children, whatever their main activity, than heads of hospital units. They also talked to the children one-and-a-half times as frequently, and were three times less likely to *ignore or reject* the children when they were with them. Each of these differences was statistically significant. The heads of hostel units were more likely to *accept* the children than the heads of hospital wards, and when they were engaged in Administrative or Domestic duties they were more likely to do these in front of the children.

Sisters and charge nurses were more likely to carry out their Domestic and Administrative tasks away from the children.

TABLE 13.4 *Performance of activities by head of unit: hostels and hospitals*[a]

| Item | 1 Hostels x̄ | SD | 2 Hospitals x̄ | SD | Differences 1–2 | t | p< |
|---|---|---|---|---|---|---|---|
| Children present | 78 | 13 | 59 | 14 | +9 | 2·35 | 0·05 |
| Staff talked | 90 | 5 | 64 | 11 | +26 | 5·29 | 0·001 |
| Evaluation: Reject | 10 | 5 | 32 | 9 | −22 | 5·52 | 0·001 |
| Evaluation: Tolerate | 56 | 11 | 50 | 11 | +6 | 0·84 | NS |
| Evaluation: Accept | 34 | 12 | 18 | 16 | +16 | 2·13 | NS |
| % of domestic and Admin. activity with interaction | 39 | 16 | 25 | 11 | +14 | 1·75 | NS |

[a] Means (x̄), standard deviation (SD) and differences have been rounded to nearest whole number. The bases for calculating children present, staff talked, evaluation, and proportion of Domestic and Administrative activity with interaction are given in the notes to Table 13.3. Degrees of freedom = 11.

Again, we looked at the hostels and hospitals separately to see if the relationship between the performance of the person in charge and the patterns of management in the unit held good within institutional types. In spite of the small numbers involved, most of the correlations were in the expected direction and in two cases reached statistical significance. Within the hospitals there was a negative correlation between the proportion of intervals in which the head of the unit was rated as *rejecting* the children and the scores on the revised Child Management Scale ($r = -0.925$, $p < 0.05$). Within the hostels there was a significant association between the amount of Domestic and Administrative activity which unit heads carried out together with the children and scale scores ($r = 0.89$, $p < 0.01$).

Together, these data provided considerable support for Hypothesis IX, that the role performance of heads of units will be related to the patterns of management obtaining in their units.

*Hypothesis X*

Following our view that household organization is associated with child-oriented patterns of care, whereas more formalized organizational structures are associated with institutionally-oriented patterns, we predicted that there would be differences between units in the way in which activities were allocated to different grades of staff. According to Hypothesis X (p. 123), we expected to find a greater diffusion of activities among senior and junior staff in child-oriented units and a greater specificity of activities, with tasks being distributed along status lines, in institutionally-oriented units. That is to say, when the activities of different grades of staff are compared, there will be greater similarities between grades in the child-oriented units than in the institutionally-oriented units.

Data on the activities of the child care status group—trained and untrained nurses in the hospitals and deputy and assistant housemothers in the hostels—are presented in Table 13.5. That data were collected from the observational studies in exactly the same way as for the heads of units.

TABLE 13.5   *Activities of child care staff: hostels and hospitals*[a]

| | 1 | | 2 | | | | |
| Activity | Hostels | | Hospitals | | Differences | t | p< |
| | $\bar{x}$ | SD | $\bar{x}$ | SD | 1–2 | | |
|---|---|---|---|---|---|---|---|
| Social Child Care | 19 | 8 | 10 | 5 | +9 | 2·09 | NS |
| Physical Child Care | 40 | 14 | 48 | 7 | −7 | 1·06 | NS |
| Supervisory Child Care | 30 | 8 | 29 | 11 | +1 | 0·13 | NS |
| Domestic duties | 27 | 8 | 22 | 2 | +5 | 1·25 | NS |
| Administration | 3 | 3 | 6 | 1 | −3 | 2·32 | 0·05 |
| Social + Physical + Supervisory | 90 | 13 | 87 | 5 | +3 | 0·44 | NS |
| Domestic + Administrative | 30 | 10 | 28 | 2 | +2 | 0·37 | NS |

[a]Means ($\bar{x}$), standard deviations (SD) and differences have been rounded to nearest whole number. Columns do not add up to 100 because more than one activity could occur in each time interval (see text). Degrees of freedom = 11.

It is apparent from Table 13.5 that junior child care staff perform substantially the same activities, and in about the same proportions, *whether they work in hostels or hospitals*. In both kinds of establishment, they spend most of their time on the Physical Care of children, followed by Supervisory activities, Domestic Duties and Social Care of the children. Only in the area of Administration was there a statistically significant difference between the two groups, with hospital staff twice as likely to be engaged in this as hostel staff (t=2·32, p<0·05). However, in both hostels and hospitals, Administration accounted for much the smallest part of the time of junior staff. When the proportions of time spent in Social, Physical and Supervisory Care are combined, and contrasted with the totals for Domestic and Administrative activities, it is clear that junior staff were virtually interchangeable between units —at least in so far as they were required to do much the same things. (We shall see later, however, that *the way they carried out* these activities differed significantly.)

We have already seen, in Table 13.2, that the activities of heads of units in hostels and hospitals were significantly different in all respects, except the amount of time spent on Domestic Duties and the Physical Care of children. To test the present Hypothesis, therefore, we need to compare the activities of heads of units and child care staff to see if there are greater similarities between the grades in the more child-oriented hostels than there are in the more institutionally-oriented hospitals. The data from Tables 13.2 and 13.5 are presented in the form of histograms in Figure 13.1 to facilitate the comparison.

It can be seen from inspection of Figure 13.1 that the pattern of activities for child care staff in hostels closely resembles the pattern for the heads of their units, whereas in the hospital units the patterns for these two status groups are quite different. Although there are statistically significant differences between hostel heads and their junior staff in Physical Child Care ($t = 3.30$, $p < 0.01$, $df = 14$) and in Administration ($t = 3.13$, $p < 0.01$, $df = 14$), it is apparent that both grades are involved in most activities to approximately the same degree. The differences between status groups in the hospital units are much greater: Physical Child Care ($t = 5.80$, $p < 0.01$, $df = 8$) is delegated for the most part to junior staff, as is Supervision ($t = 2.26$, $p < 0.10$, $df = 8$), while Administration is carried out by the senior staff ($t = 6.21$, $p < 0.01$, $df = 8$).

When we combined Social, Physical and Supervisory Child Care on the one hand, and Domestic and Administrative activity on the other, and then compared status groups, the similarities between groups in hostels, and the differences in hospitals, were very marked. The results are presented in Table 13.6.

Further support for these findings was derived from a different source. On Form C4 Appendix II, pp. 227–30), we invited all members of staff to record whether they undertook any activities, from a representative check list, as part of their normal duties or not. The check list contained items from our observational check list, and covered Domestic and Administrative activities as well as the various aspects of Child Care. The responses of unit heads and child care staff were compared in each of these areas, in hostels and in hospitals. Activities were regarded as common to both status groups if both the head of the unit and 50 per cent of

169

M

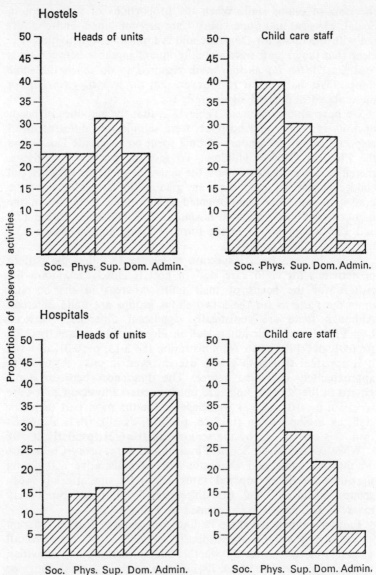

Fig. 13.1 *Staff activities in hostels and hospitals*

the child care staff claimed normally to undertake the activity. The proportion of activities which were common to both status groups was significantly higher than in the hospitals, where more activities were specific to one or the other status group ($t = 2 \cdot 87$, $p < 0 \cdot 02$, df $= 11$).

TABLE 13.6   *Mean activities of head of unit and child care staff: hostels and hospitals*[a]

|  | 1 Head of unit | | 2 C.C. staff | | Differences | | | |
| --- | --- | --- | --- | --- | --- | --- | --- | --- |
|  | $\bar{x}$ | SD | $\bar{x}$ | SD | 1–2 | t | df | p< |
| *Hostels* | | | | | | | | |
| Social + Physical + Supervisory Child Care | 77 | 17 | 90 | 13 | −13 | 1·76 | 14 | NS |
| Domestic + Administrative | 36 | 15 | 30 | 10 | +6 | 0·90 | 14 | NS |
| *Hospitals* | | | | | | | | |
| Social + Physical + Supervisory Child Care | 40 | 15 | 87 | 5 | −47 | 5·00 | 8 | 0·002 |
| Domestic + Administrative | 63 | 12 | 28 | 2 | +35 | 6·43 | 8 | 0·001 |

[a]Means ($\bar{x}$), standard deviations (SD), and differences rounded to nearest whole number. Columns do not add up to 100 because more than one activity could occur in each time interval (see text).

*Hypothesis XI*

According to Hypothesis XI (p. 124), we predicted that junior staff in child-oriented units would, like their seniors, interact with the children in a way characterized by greater warmth and a greater frequency of talk than their counterparts in institutionally-oriented units. That is, we expected the role performance of junior staff to follow the pattern of role performance for senior staff in their units. We have already seen, from Table 13.5, that there were scarcely any major differences in the activities that junior staff were required to carry out when hostels and hospitals were compared. Nonetheless, there were significant differences in the way junior staff performed their duties in the different types of establishment. The data are presented in Table 13.7.

Not surprisingly, there was little difference in the amount of contact junior staff had with children, since about three-quarters of their activities were of various kinds of child care, which necessarily involved them with children. But on the occasions when junior staff were with children, hostel staff were significantly more likely to be talking to the children ($t=2\cdot62$, $p<0\cdot05$) and significantly less likely to act towards them in a *rejecting* manner ($t=2\cdot81$, $p<0\cdot02$) than hospital staff. Although these differences are

171

less marked than those between heads of units in the two types of institution, the hypothesis that junior staff in the child-oriented units would be warmer in their dealings with the children, and talk to them more frequently, is confirmed.

TABLE 13.7 *Performance of activities by child care staff: hostels and hospitals*[a]

| Item | 1 Hostels $\bar{x}$ | SD | 2 Hospitals $\bar{x}$ | SD | Differences 1–2 | t | p< |
|---|---|---|---|---|---|---|---|
| Children present | 91 | 8 | 93 | 3 | −2 | 0·56 | NS |
| Staff talked | 84 | 9 | 69 | 10 | +15 | 2·62 | 0·05 |
| Reject | 12 | 6 | 26 | 11 | −14 | 2·81 | 0·02 |
| Evaluation: Tolerate | 59 | 12 | 58 | 9 | +1 | 0·15 | NS |
| Accept | 28 | 15 | 15 | 10 | +13 | 1·58 | NS |

[a]Means ($\bar{x}$), standard deviations (SD), and differences have been rounded to nearest whole number. The bases for calculating children present, staff talked, and evaluation proportions are the same as for heads of units – see notes to Table 13.3. Degrees of freedom = 11.

## The importance of the head of the unit's role

The way in which the role performance of junior staff in hospitals and hostels mirrors the role performance of senior staff in their respective units, suggests that the unit head—sister or superintendent—is a key figure in establishing and maintaining the patterns of staff behaviour for her unit. We examine some of the factors which might influence the role of the head of the unit in the next chapter. But what are the implications of the different patterning of staff roles in different situations?

At the end of the field studies (see Chapter 8) we suggested that the superior abilities in feeding and speech of the children in the Local Authority hostel and the voluntary home, when compared with an otherwise similar group of children in the hospital ward, might be attributable to the management practices in the different environments. In particular, we pointed to the fact that meal-times were not social occasions in the hospital ward, and that staff did not eat with the children who, in consequence, had no adult model to follow. It was also our impression, though we had no 'hard' data in this area, that the staff in the hospital ward spoke less frequently to the children, and with less warmth, than staff in the other types of unit. The findings from the survey, and particularly from the study of staff role performance, amply confirm these impressions. It is therefore interesting to see whether differences in speech, feeding and other skills are to be found among the children in the survey in a way that is related to the role performance of the staff in their units.

It should be stressed that our findings here, from cross-sectional data, do not constitute a test of any hypothesis linking staff role performance to the skills of the children in their care. Selective factors cannot be ruled out as a possible explanation for any differences. Nonetheless, the results suggest that further investigation would be worthwhile. In order to reduce the possible influence of selective factors to a minimum, we limited our comparison to closely comparable groups of children with the same diagnosis and similar degrees of mental defect and physical impairment. We examined only Mongol children aged five years or over, who had IQs of 30 points or more, who were fully ambulant and who had no physical disabilities other than those directly associated with Down's syndrome.* For the purposes of analysis, the children of this type in the voluntary homes were combined with those in the hostels. There were 29 such children in the hospitals and 39 in the hostels and voluntary homes.

TABLE 13.8    *Feeding skills of Mongols*[a]

|  | N | Use knife and fork | Use spoon | Require more help or fed |
|---|---|---|---|---|
| Hospitals | 29 | 9 | 16 | 4 |
| Hostels and voluntary homes | 39 | 31 | 5 | 3 |

[a]Mongols aged five years or more, with IQs more than 30 points, who were ambulant and had no physical disabilities.

TABLE 13.9    *Verbal skills of Mongols*[a]

|  | N | Use sentences | Use isolated words only | No intelligible speech |
|---|---|---|---|---|
| Hospitals | 29 | 10 | 11 | 8 |
| Hostels and voluntary homes | 39 | 30 | 8 | 1 |

[a]Mongols aged five years or more, with IQs more than 30 points, who were ambulant and had no physical disabilities.

* Similar trends were found when the age groups 5–10, 10–14 and 15+ years were examined, but the numbers were too small to apply satisfactory statistical tests.

The Mongols in the hostels and voluntary homes were significantly more advanced in feeding than those in the hospitals ($x^2 = 16\cdot90$, df = 2, $p < 0\cdot001$). Table 13.8 presents the data.

Much the same pattern was found in respect of speech. Significantly more of the Mongols in the voluntary homes and the hostels were able to use sentences than those in the hospitals ($x^2 = 14\cdot77$, df = 2, $p < 0\cdot001$). The results are given in Table 13·9.

There were no significant differences between the groups of Mongols with regard to their abilities in dressing, degrees of incontinence and the prevalence of behaviour disorders.

# 14 The responsibility and training of senior staff

We have now examined a number of hypotheses derived from the more general view that 'householdness' is associated with child-oriented patterns of care. In the last chapter we discussed the activities of different status groups, and it was suggested, on the evidence presented there, that the role of the person in charge of each unit was critical for setting the pattern in that unit. The more unit heads were involved in the everyday care and supervision of the children, and the more they talked with them, the more likely were junior staff to behave warmly towards their charges, and the more child-oriented were the patterns of care in the unit.

For the most part, the findings showed that just as there were two patterns of care—a hostel pattern and a hospital pattern—so there were two patterns of staff activities. However, on some variables it was possible to show differences within hostels and differences within hospitals which were related to the patterns of care in the predicted directions. Because scores on the variables we studied were highly intercorrelated, and because only a small number of establishments was surveyed, it is not possible to say whether this picture of two distinct types of institutional treatment has been produced by one factor rather than another. Almost certainly, a number of factors are involved. We pointed out, however, that our findings did not reflect on individual members of staff. Instead, we suggested that individual differences were outweighed by broader, structural constraints—the administrative organization within which staff operated and the training programmes which were designed to support their work. In the present chapter we discuss the evidence in relation to these matters.

There are many standpoints from which the administrative

organization of the institutions could be viewed. We decided to study one aspect which seemed to be closely related to our conception of households, namely, the amount of responsibility delegated to, and exercised by, the unit head. In the community, households are autonomous units making their own decisions: how they come to decisions may vary from household to household, and from one type of decision to another, but in our society decisions are usually made from a number of possible choices, and the household or the householder is held responsible for the decisions reached. Where the units of an institution were relatively autonomous, and a high degree of responsibility was vested in the unit head, we expected to find a lack of status distinctions in the activities of staff, with heads of units as well as junior staff involved in the everyday care of children. We also expected to find a child-oriented pattern of care.

Before describing the way we assessed the responsibility of senior staff and the autonomy of their units, something should be said about the place which the units occupied in the wider organizational structures of which they were part. Although the heads of all units had some responsibility for the day-to-day running of their affairs, all units were parts of more or less complex hierarchical structures, the nature of which had implications for the role of the unit head.

Each of the hospital wards was physically part of a set of similar wards grouped within a defined area, and was organizationally integrated within the tripartite medical, nursing and administrative structure of the hospital, similar to that outlined in Chapter 6. Each ward was dependent for many of its goods and services on the departments outside the unit which served the whole hospital. Ward sisters and charge nurses had superiors in both the medical and the nursing hierarchies, and were expected to co-operate with many departments in a complex system of organization. Above all, the hospitals were linked by certain traditions, embodied in the medical and nursing *professions,* and by administrative arrangements which made them part of a common *hospital service.*

The units in the voluntary homes were integrated into a rather different kind of organizational structure. Each was physically part of a larger complex of units, although typically the boundaries of these units were less clearly marked than those for hospital wards. Units frequently shared various common facilities. There were no separate hierarchies in the voluntary homes, nor were there many departments with specialized functions. Most of the administration was carried out on the site, there being little in the way of head office control, except over broad financial matters. Typically, a small administrative staff exercised a general supervision of the living units, and they dealt with a great many matters, either at the request of the units or as a matter of routine. The relationship between the administration and the units was, in some cases, paternalistic; in others, autocratic. Although two of the homes had well-established traditions of care and were linked to other institutions run by the same society, none had the kind of wider professional and administrative network that characterized the hospitals.

The hostel units presented several different patterns, but all of them formed part of the Department of Health in particular Local Authorities. Seven of the eight were physically separate units and only one was physically linked with another, identical unit. All of them, however, were situated near, or in the same grounds as, a training centre which children from the hostels attended. In five of the hostels we studied, the head of the unit was directly responsible to officers in the Department of Health of the Local Authority—through the mental welfare officers, to the Deputy Medical Officer of Health, or in some cases to various other senior officers in the Health Department. In the remaining three hostels, the head of the unit was responsible to a warden who worked on the same site, and who in turn was responsible for both the hostel and the training centre to the appropriate officers in the Local Health Authority.

Most of the hostels were partly dependent upon service personnel who were not exclusively concerned with the day-to-day running of the hostel: for example, one hostel had a cook who prepared meals for the children in the training centre as well as children resident in the hostel. Moreover, all the hostels were dependent on outside bodies for some of their services, such as welfare services and medical services, which were obtained from local general practitioners. There was little that could be termed a 'tradition' in the way the hostels were run, or in the professional background of staff, and few of the Local Authorities at that time had more than one hostel. Indeed, we found that many staff felt professionally isolated.* We formed the impression that the work of the Children's Departments had to some extent provided a model for some hostels, and many Authorities sought their staff from among

* We made no direct study of the attitudes of staff or their feelings about their work, although many of our respondents talked about these matters. Inevitably, many people asked the research workers for opinions, and even recommendations about the care of the subnormal and the organization of their units. These enquiries were much more marked among hostel staff, and it was only in relation to hostels that this curiosity was also found at an administrative level, for example among mental welfare officers. This suggests a greater isolation from professional supports among those concerned in Local Authority hostels.

those who had received their training or previous experience in residential nurseries or children's homes.

## Hypothesis XII

In Hypothesis XII (p. 124) we argued that the activities of heads of units will be related to the amount of responsibility they are given within the wider organization of the institution. In particular, we predicted that unit heads will be *more* involved in personal child care when they have a personal responsibility for *more* aspects of the unit's functioning, than when they are 'relieved' of such duties and responsibilities by superordinate staff.

It will be recalled from Chapter 9 that we proposed to assess the autonomy of units, and the responsibility of the unit heads, by (1) the degree of freedom from inspection and supervision by superiors which she enjoyed; and by the degree of control she had over (2) policy decisions affecting the children, (3) buying goods for the children and the unit, (4) staffing decisions and (5) matters relating to unit management, particularly the organization of the children's regimen. We asked questions of the head of each unit about each of these areas of responsibility, using Form C3 (see Appendix II, pp. 223–6).

## Inspections of the unit

One index of the amount of control exercised over the unit is the number of inspections of it which are made by superiors. The more frequent the visits of inspection by superiors, the greater the likelihood that they will directly influence the management of the unit and thus curtail the responsibility of the unit head.

All units were visited by superior 'line' staff (that is, in the hospitals, by the matron or an assistant matron who was higher in rank than the ward sister, and in the hostels by a senior welfare officer or an administrative officer occupying an analogous position), but the visits differed markedly in frequency. Hospital units were visited, on average, 18·2 times per week: one was visited four times a day, one three times a day and the remaining three units twice daily. Hostel units, on the other hand, received an average of 1·4 visits per week: one was inspected on a daily basis, three units were visited weekly, while four hostels were visited only once a month. In the voluntary homes, one was inspected three times a day, one daily and the third weekly. If, as we suspect, unit autonomy is incompatible with frequent visits of inspection, one would expect to find much less responsibility formally assigned to the heads of hospital units than to the heads of the hostel units.

## Areas of responsibility

The questions in each of the areas of possible responsibility given to unit heads were designed so that responses could be scored on a three-point scale: a score of 0 was given when the unit head was judged to have little or no discretion in the matter, a score of 1 indicated some degree of responsibility and a score of 2 was given only when she approached the degree of responsibility which might be expected for an ordinary householder in the community. Examples of the ratings are given below. For each type of unit we first compared the proportions of responses scoring 0, 1 and 2 in each of the areas of responsibility and then, for those areas which discriminated between units, we treated the questions as though they were items on a scale, and the scores were summed to give a simple index of responsibility for each unit.

## Policy decisions affecting the children

The unit heads were asked to describe who was involved and what part each person played in deciding a number of policy matters in relation to children. Specifically, they were asked about who decided which children were (1) admitted to the unit; (2) discharged from the unit; (3) ready to attend school; (4) requiring specialist treatment. Scores were assigned as follows. Responses that indicated that unit heads were not involved were given a score of 0. Responses which indicated that the head of the unit was involved in discussion about the matter, the actual decision resting finally with a superior or specialist, were scored 1. Responses which indicated that the unit head planned events, with or without prior consultation with other people, and was responsible for the final decision about them, were scored 2.

In none of the units was the unit head responsible for making a final decision about any of these four matters. In all cases, the decisions were taken by specialist staff, although unit heads were sometimes consulted on some of them.* There were thus no scores of 2 awarded, and the distribution of scores of 0 and 1 did not systematically discriminate between units. There was no evidence,

---

* Legal considerations play a part here. All policy decisions involve an answer to the question, 'Who has the right to make them?' Frequently, wider values are involved in this, beyond the immediate considerations of organizational efficiency. The problem of authorizing decisions, Parsons (1960, p. 31) tells us, 'connects with the value system [of society] and hence with the problem of legitimacy'. Nowhere is this more likely to be true than in the care of decisions affecting children in public care. In our society, there is a strong tradition (and demand) that such decisions are taken by qualified medical or other professionals or by publicly accountable officers.

therefore, to support our view that responsibility for policy matters relating to the children would be related to the patterns of care. Since these items did not discriminate between units, they were eliminated from the Responsibility Index.

### The acquisition of goods for the unit

The unit head was asked to describe how she obtained clothing and toys, groceries, greengroceries and bread, linen and crockery, soft furnishings and cleaning materials for use in the unit. There were nine questions, one for each type of article. Responses which were scored 0 included the routine supply of clothes to the unit, graded roughly according to size only, and situations in which an order form, completed by the head of the unit, had to be submitted to at least one superior for approval before it could be complied with by the store or department which supplied the goods. Examples of responses graded 1 were those found in a number of establishments in which the head of the unit would complete an order for foodstuffs and send it directly to a central supplies department, which would deliver the goods directly to her. Such procedures limited her discretion less obviously than those which we grouped in the first category, but the prescription that she used a central supplier with no alternative source open to her still involved some formal curtailment of the extent of her choice.

In the third category were grouped the procedures in which the head of the unit sent her orders direct to an outside supplier whom she had either chosen herself, or who was one of a number of firms specified by the authorities. These arrangements meant that the head of the unit might go to a number of shops in her area. At these, she might either use a cash allowance or a credit system which had been agreed between the authorities and the retailer. (There were, in fact, very few instances of unit heads being given a cash allowance for their purchases, although in six units, one hospital and five hostels, the unit's head had a petty cash allowance.)

There were marked differences between institutions of different types in the amount of responsibility given to heads of units on these matters. The mean frequency of scores of 0, 1 and 2 was, for the hospitals, 7·8, 1, 0·2; for voluntary homes it was 6, 1·7, 1·3; and for the hostels 3, 1·6, 4·4. That is, the average frequency of scores of 2, representing maximum choice, was twenty times as great in the hostels as it was in the hospitals, and the average frequency for scores of 0, representing procedures which meant that the head of the unit had no discretion in obtaining these items, was two-and-a-half times as great in the hospitals and twice as high in the voluntary homes as it was in the hostels.

## The arrangement of matters relating to the staff in the unit

Unit heads were asked to describe procedures by which off duty for the week was arranged; holidays for staff were allocated; tasks in the unit were allocated; and the new staff were appointed. In all of the units, the allocation of jobs to staff was the exclusive responsibility of the head of the unit. Thus, there were only three items for which there was any variation between units. A score of 0 was given when the head of the unit was not involved in these arrangements; a score of 1 was given is she was consulted before the decision was made; and if she made the arrangements without the need to consult superiors or specialists, a score of 2 was assigned.

In only one hostel and on only one of the three items was the head of the unit not involved with the arrangements concerned with the staffing of her unit. By contrast, in four out of the five wards, the ward sisters were not involved at all in such arrangements. In none of the wards were they involved in making arrangements for off duty or for the appointment of new staff to work in a ward. In two of the voluntary homes, unit heads had no powers in arranging one of the three items they were asked about. The average frequency of scores of 0, 1 and 2 respectively for the hospitals was 1·8, 0·2, 1; for the voluntary homes 0·7, 1·6, 0·7; and for the hostels 0·1, 1·1, 1·8. Thus, despite the small number of items, the same pattern was found as that shown from the question about the amount of responsibility given to the unit head in the acquisition of goods.

## Unit management and the children's regimen

To ascertain what degree of discretion the unit head had in this area, we asked if, in her planning of the routine, she was limited by the existence of rules laid down by superior authorities. Specifically, the unit heads were asked if there were rules relating to the following aspects of the children's routine, or if the unit heads were free to make their own decisions about them: getting-up times; bed-times; toileting times; meal-times; visiting times; the number of baths the children had.

A score of 0 indicated the existence of a rule which allowed no discretion; a score of 1 was given when the rule was either permissive or merely defined general limits within which the unit head could plan as she wished; a score of 2 was assigned when the unit head was not bound by rules in the matter in question.

The average frequency of the scores of 0, 1 and 2 respectively for the hospitals was 2·4, 2·0 and 1·6; for the voluntary homes it was 2·7, 1·3 and 2·0; and for the hostels 0·1, 0·0 and 5·9. Thus,

**181**

the average frequency of scores of 2 was four times as high in the hostels as it was in the hospitals and twice as high as it was in the voluntary homes. Once again, the same pattern emerged as between units of different types.

## An index of responsibility

The data reported above strongly suggest that, whereas heads of units in hostels are largely responsible for the day-to-day running of affairs in their units, the effective responsibilities for much of the daily management in the hospitals and voluntary homes are assumed by superiors. These differences emerge very strikingly when the scores obtained by each of the units in these areas are added together to form a Responsibility Index. There are eighteen items which yield a range of scores from 0 to 36, high scores indicating a high degree of responsibility for the unit head. Figure 14.1 presents the results.

There was no overlap between the scores of the hostels and hospitals, and the differences between the means were highly significant statistically. The mean and standard deviation for the hospitals were 8·8 and 5·2 respectively, and for the hostels 26·1 and 2·2 ($t=12\cdot38$, $p<0\cdot001$, $df=11$). We have already seen that there was no overlap between the hostels and the hospitals in scores on the revised Child Management Scale, and that the heads of the hostel units were more personally involved in the Social, Physical and Supervisory Care of the children, so that these data provide general confirmation of Hypothesis XII.

There were also statistically significant rank order correlations, all in the predicted directions, between scores on the Responsibility Index and the amount of time that heads of units spent in various activities (Social Child Care, $r=0\cdot48$, $p<0\cdot05$; Supervisory Child Care, $r=0\cdot50$, $p<0\cdot5$; Domestic and Administrative activities, $r=-0\cdot46$, $p<0\cdot05$; and amount of talk, $r=0\cdot65$, $p<0\cdot05$), but to a large extent these simply reflect the differences already referred to between hostels and hospitals.

When hostels and hospitals were looked at as separate groups, there were no systematic relationships between Responsibility scores and the other variables, possibly because the variance within each of these groups was very small. It is instructive, however, to examine the three voluntary homes in this respect. Figure 14·1 shows that two of the voluntary homes fall within the range of scores of the hospitals on the Responsibility Index, while the third is more than one standard deviation above the highest score of any hospital ward. The scores of the three units of the voluntary homes on the revised Child Management Scale decrease (i.e become

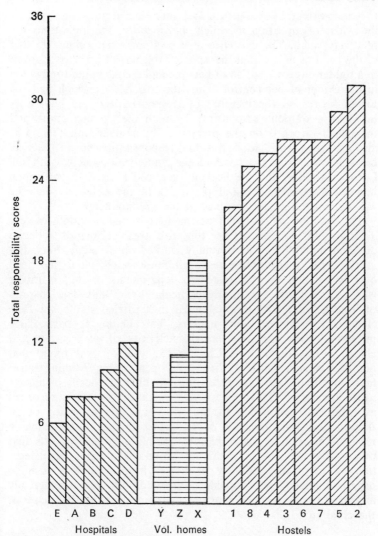

Fig. 14.1 *A Responsibility Index*

more child-oriented) as the amount of responsibility of the unit head, as measured by this index, increases.

The data indicate that the term 'unit head', which we have used throughout these studies, takes on a quite different significance in different organizational settings. In the hostels, the position of the head of the unit does not merely carry status, but also effective control over a wide range of unit matters. In each unit there is only one person in charge, and although her authority is limited

183

to some extent by budgeting and other constraints imposed by the wider organization in which she operates, the limitations are relatively small. The existence of a position superordinate to that of the head of unit within the same establishment appears to result in a tighter circumscription of her role and a concomitant reduction in the extent of her control. Thus the two hostels which had the lowest scores on the measure of Responsibility were both ones in which a warden—responsible for both the training centre and the hostel—worked on the premises. (In another unit there was also a warden who had such a dual responsibility, but in practice, his wife, who was the head of the unit, dealt directly with the Local Authority, and the husband confined himself to gardening, household maintenance and playing with the children when he was not professionally occupied at the training centre.)

The position of the head of the unit in the hospitals is very different. In two instances, this role was performed by two different individuals who normally worked on different shifts. But in all wards, many of the responsibilities which fell to the head of a hostel unit were entrusted to departments or staff members who were not attached to any particular living unit. The position of head of unit in a hospital ward thus carried status but little effective control over unit matters. This finding is particularly intriguing when one considers the activities of ward sisters and charge nurses reported in Chapter 13, where it was found that not only was a third of their time spent doing Administrative tasks, but that they were three times as likely as heads of hostels to be so engaged. This suggests that much of the activity recorded as Administrative within the hospitals was administration of an *intermediary kind required by the wider organization*—filling in requisitions, writing daily reports, maintaining records—so that others whose responsibility this was could check them. The delegation of more responsibility to hostel heads, allowing them to negotiate directly with outsiders for goods and services, actually appears to have released more of their time for the daily care of the children.

## Hypothesis XIII

The second factor we chose to examine in seeking an explanation for the differences in the patterns of staff activities, and more particularly the way those activities were performed, was staff training. No doubt there are many influences on the way staff perform their roles—age, marital status, general health, intelligence, beliefs, personality and other physical and psychological factors. We made no systematic study of these, partly because our interests were more specifically sociological, and partly because such demographic and psychological characteristics would be better examined in a different kind of study, with rather larger numbers.*

Information about type of training was obtained by questionnaire (Form C4, p. 227), which staff posted back to the research unit in London after the fieldwork was completed. All the unit heads returned their questionnaires, and of the 136 junior staff employed in the 16 units during the weeks of the survey, 118 replied. For analysis purposes, we divided type of training into three categories: nurse training, child care training (with or without nurse training as well), and no relevant training. Nurse training included three-year courses leading to registration in the Nursing of Sick Children (R.S.C.N.) and the Nursing of the Mentally Subnormal (R.N.M.S.) as well as general nursing and the two-year training leading to State Enrolment (S.E.N.). Child care training included Home Office and other university courses in child care, lasting not more than one year; diploma courses for teachers of the mentally handicapped which, in the case of the four hostel staff who possessed such diplomas, also lasted for one year; and a number of in-service training courses organized by Local Authorities. The manner in which staff had been trained is set out in Table 14.1.

All but one of the heads of units had received a relevant course of professional training. The seven nursing sisters or charge nurses (there were two wards which had two persons in charge, working on alternate shifts) were trained in mental subnormality nursing, and two were also trained in general nursing. Three of the heads of hostel units were nurse trained and five had received child care training. Of the heads of units in the voluntary homes, one was nurse trained, one child care trained and one had received no training at all.

A high proportion of junior staff were untrained in all types of establishment. Because of the high non-response rate among junior nurses in the hospitals (22 out of 69, or 32 per cent), there is some uncertainty about the proportion of nurses who were trained, or

---

* Over two-fifths of the staff in both hostels and hospitals were married, as were one-third in the voluntary homes. In the hostels, there were 31 per cent of staff under 25 years, while the proportion for hospitals was 18 per cent and 75 per cent in the voluntary homes. Only 4 per cent of the staff in the hospitals, and none in the voluntary homes, were aged more than 55 years, compared to 29 per cent in the hostels. About half the unit heads in hospitals were between the ages of 35 and 44, the remainder being equally divided between those aged 25 to 34 and those aged 45 to 54. Half the unit heads in hostels were between 55 and 64, and none of them was aged less than 35 years. Two of the unit heads in the voluntary homes were between 25 and 34, and one was between 45 and 54 years.

185

o

TABLE 14.1 *Percentages of staff with different trainings in sixteen institutions*[a]

|  | Nurse training | Child care training | None relevant | No information |
|---|---|---|---|---|
| *Heads of units* | | | | |
| Hospitals[b] (N = 7) | 100 | 0 | 0 | 0 |
| Hostels (N = 8) | 38 | 63 | 0 | 0 |
| Voluntary homes (N = 3) | 33 | 33 | 33 | 0 |
| Total (N = 18) | 61 | 33 | 6 | 0 |
| *Junior staff* | | | | |
| Hospitals (N = 69) | 22 | 1 | 45 | 32 |
| Hostels (N = 40) | 20 | 13 | 67 | 0 |
| Voluntary homes (N = 9) | 0 | 0 | 89 | 11 |
| Total (N = 118) | 19 | 5 | 57 | 20 |

[a] Figures rounded to nearest whole number.
[b] Two hospital units had two heads of units working on alternate shifts.

in training, in the hospital units. Judging from the hospital units where the response rate was highest, and also from the hospitals examined in the field studies, it is thought that the proportion of untrained staff would not be higher than that for the hostels, where two-thirds of the junior staff were untrained. It is unlikely, therefore, that the differences in staff roles and the patterns of care could be accounted for simply in terms of the proportions of trained and untrained staff. It is rather to the appropriateness of different types of training that one must look for explanations.

Because so many junior staff in all types of unit were untrained, we restricted any further analysis to the heads of units—a status group which, as we have already argued, seemed in any case to be of overriding importance in determining events in the living units.

According to Hypothesis XIII (p. 124), we predicted that the role performance of unit heads would be related to the training they had received in the following way. We expected that unit heads who have high rates of interaction with the children would have received a training in 'child care' in which such matters are given some emphasis; and that unit heads with low rates of interaction would have been trained as nurses, with a primary emphasis on the physical aspects of health and disease.

We found considerable support for this hypothesis. Since the role performance of staff has already been shown to be related to the patterns of child management in living units, we first related the training of heads of units to scores on the revised Child Management Scale. The data are presented graphically in Figure 14.2.

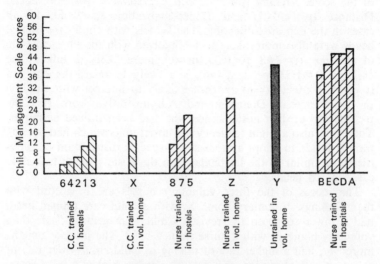

Fig. 14.2 *Training of unit heads and Child Management Scale Scores*

The training of staff was one of the few variables in which there was an overlap between institutions of different types. There were significant differences between units having nursing trained heads (5 hospitals, 3 hostels and 1 voluntary home) and units having child care trained heads (5 hostels and 1 voluntary home) in relation to Child Management Scale scores (t=3·97, p<0·01, df=13). There were also significant differences between these two groups in relation to three of the measures of role performance discussed in Chapter 13. Child care trained heads were more likely to talk to children (t=2·78, p<0·02, df=13); less likely to *reject* children (t=2·90, p<0·02, df=13); and more likely to be interacting with children while engaged on Domestic or Administrative duties (t=3·36, p<0·01, df=13) than heads of units who were nurse trained. The voluntary home with an untrained unit head was excluded from this analysis.

Not only were these differences found when all institutions were considered, but *the same general pattern was found within the hostels, and within the voluntary homes where the unit heads had been differently trained*. The five hostels in which the head was child care trained had an average revised Child Management Scale score of 7·4, whereas the three units in which the head was nurse trained had a mean score of 17·0. Despite the small size of the samples, this difference is statistically significant ($t=2·61$, $p <0·05$, $df=6$). These differences were manifested in all four parts of the scale, *Rigidity* ($p=NS$), *'Block Treatment'* ($p<0.1$), Social Distance ($p=<0·01$) and Depersenalization ($p<0·05$), in all cases in the expected direction. The hostels with child care trained heads were also more likely to be involved with the Physical Care of children, ($t=2·48$, $p<0·05$, $df=6$), more likely to talk to the children ($t=1·53$, $p<2$, $df=6$), less likely to *reject* the children ($t=1·51$, $p<0·2$, $df=6$) and more likely to interact with children in the course of Domestic and Administrative work ($t=2·06$, $p<0·1$, $df=6$) than hostel heads who had been trained as nurses. There was also a slight tendency for hostel units which had nursing trained heads to adopt a more status-specific distribution of activities (i.e. similar to the hospitals) than the hostels which had child care trained heads.

The scores of the three voluntary homes are in accord with these findings. Voluntary home X, with a child care trained head, had a lower score on the revised Child Management Scale than voluntary home Z, with a nurse trained head. The head of unit X, moreover, had a higher rate of talking to children, a lower rate of *rejection*, a higher rate of *acceptance* and a higher rate of interaction during Domestic and Administrative work, than the head of unit Z—as can be seen from Table 13.3 in the previous chapter. Voluntary home Y, with a head of unit who had received no relevant training, resembled the hospital units in a great many respects, including the pattern of role performance of the person in charge.

We should make it clear that we have made no detailed analysis of the content of different training programmes. None-the-less, these findings suggest that the type of training received by staff exercises a powerful influence—not only on the way in which they carry out their duties, but also on the patterns of care maintained in their units. Within the broad constraints imposed by the organizational structure of establishments of different types—hostels, hospitals and voluntary homes—the training of unit heads seems to be a most important variable in determining what happens within the units.

# part four

# Conclusions

# 15   Summary and conclusions

In this monograph we have reported a series of studies in institutions for handicapped children. The aims of our enquiries were first to describe characteristic patterns of child management in different institutions; second, to find ways of quantifying these patterns to facilitate systematic comparisons between institutions; and third, to try to account for any differences in the methods of upbringing in sociological terms.

We have been concerned only with longstay institutions, and for the most part we have confined our attention to institutions for retarded children. It is in that field that our findings, therefore, should have the most practical impact. But from the outset our interest was theoretical as well as practical, and we approached our subject matter from within the framework of the sociology of residential organizations. To the extent that we were successful in developing a method for measuring the dimension of inmate management, a start has been made towards the systematic study of the functioning of such institutions. But it is only a beginning. We hope that our examination of other organizational variables might provide the basis for the further dimensional analysis of the structure of residential organizations. In this concluding chapter, we seek to summarize our work, to draw attention to its limitations and to point up its implications.

The studies described here extended over a period of about four years. During this time, we looked at more than 100 separate living units in twenty-six different establishments. Our first enquiries, which we have called the *field studies,* took us into four large residential establishments; two children's homes with 22 and 36 units respectively, and two hospitals, one for subnormal children with 16 units and one for physically handicapped children in

191

which we studied 5 wards. Case studies in these establishments were followed by fieldwork in a Local Authority hostel and in a voluntary home, both of which cared for the subnormal.

Following the field studies, the methods of research were revised and developed in further pilot enquiries conducted in four more institutions, and we then carried out a *survey* of sixteen institutions for mentally retarded children, in each of which one living unit was selected for study.

The *field studies* demonstrated that there were remarkable differences in child management practices between different types of institution serving different types of children. Children in the Local Authority children's homes were brought up in a child-oriented manner which contrasted markedly with the institutionally-oriented pattern of care in the hospital for the mentally subnormal. The paediatric hospital resembled the subnormality hospital in its pattern of care more closely than it did either of the homes for deprived children. Closer investigation, however, indicated that these differences could not be plausibly attributed to the characteristics of the children. There were, for example, no systematic differences in patterns of care between low- and high-grade wards in the subnormality hospital, and there was ample evidence in the literature to suggest that non-handicapped but deprived children had been brought up in an institutionally-oriented manner in the past.

In an effort to quantify the differences in child upbringing a Child Management Scale was developed and tested in the four large institutions in which the field studies had been carried out. This scale was then applied in a Local Authority hostel, and the living units of a voluntary home, which cared for mentally retarded children similar to the children in some, but not all, of the wards of the mental subnormality hospital. Again the differences were very striking: there was no overlap in scale scores between the most institutionally-oriented of the units in the new establishments and the least institutionally-oriented of the wards in either the subnormality hospital or the paediatric hospital. Indeed, the mentally retarded children in the hostel and the voluntary home led lives which were very similar to those of the deprived children in the children's homes. In these units the children were accorded respect as individuals; they had opportunities both for privacy and companionship, for personal clothing and for a share in the possessions of the community; they lived in an environment where rules were few and exceptions to them readily made, and where the staff were friendly and had an opportunity to get to know them. In these units the staff worked for long periods of time with a single group of children. In the hospitals the needs of young children for affection, for individual treatment, for variety of experience and for continuity of relationships received little attention. Treatment was not harsh or cruel, but the environment was bleak and the atmosphere institutional.

We sought to explain the reason for these differences not in terms of the personal characteristics of the staff—whose work in difficult circumstances won our respect—but in the social organization in which staff carried out their duties. The *survey* of units in sixteen institutions for the mentally retarded was designed to quantify some aspects of organizational structure, to explore their inter-relations and especially to examine their relationship to patterns of care. Before the survey was carried out, further pilot work was undertaken in which the Child Management Scale was revised and expanded, and a number of other measuring instruments were developed.

Using the results of the field studies as a guide, we put forward a number of hypotheses, which might account for differences in the patterns of care, for testing in the survey. The term 'hypotheses' may seem rather grand for predictions which have a relatively low level of generality, even though several of them were derived from a more general proposition, namely that 'householdness' would be associated with child-oriented patterns of care. We expressed our ideas, as precisely as we could, in this way because we wished to formulate our expectations in terms that would render them falsifiable and which might facilitate replication.

Five hospitals, eight Local Authority hostels and three voluntary homes were selected for the survey, all caring for severely retarded children. We will briefly summarize the main findings in relation to each of the hypotheses, before discussing the implications of the study.

## Hypothesis 1

Our first hypothesis, that there would be large and characteristic differences in child management practices, as these were measured by the revised Child Management Scale, between the three institutional types was generally confirmed. The hostels, with mainly child-oriented patterns of care, had a mean scale score of 11 points, and the hospitals with institutionally-oriented patterns of care, had a mean score of 43 points. The mean score for the voluntary homes, however, conceals wide variations within this type: one voluntary home had a score of 14 similar to the hostels, another a score of 41 similar to the hospitals, while a third had a score of 28 intermediate between those patterns.

*Hypothesis II*

Our data in respect of the prediction that differences in management practices will not be related to the level of handicaps of the residents are difficult to interpret. In part it is a question of degree: the very large differences in handicaps between the residents in the hostel and the voluntary home for the subnormal and the homes for deprived children in the field studies did not prevent all these units having similarly child-oriented patterns of care. On the other hand, there are comparatively small but systematic differences in the level of handicaps of the residents in different types of units in the survey. The children in the hospitals were generally rather more handicapped and were brought up with more institutionally-oriented patterns of care than children in the other institutions. Even so, it was possible to find units of different types—hostels and hospitals—caring for very similar groups of children, but with dramatically different patterns of care. Moreover, when the individual items of the revised Child Management Scale are examined there is no reason to suppose that handicaps should influence any of these practices. On balance, we think that while certain types of handicaps may mean that perhaps more staff are required to maintain child-oriented patterns of care, handicaps of residents are not an overriding factor in determining child management practices.

*Hypothesis III*

Although the size of institutions was found to be related to scale scores, we found this to result from the fact that there was no overlap in size between institutions of different types. Indeed within institutional types there was a slight tendency for smaller institutions to have more institutionally-oriented patterns of care. Though we did not succeed in finding a large hospital with child-oriented patterns of care, both the large children's homes in the field studies maintained very child-oriented practices. The revised Child Management Scale, of course, measures only certain aspects of the everyday care of children, and many of the arguments for or against large institutions are concerned with other matters, but our hypothesis that management practices are not affected by institutional size was confirmed.

*Hypothesis IV*

The hypothesis that size of living units could not be related to management practices was also confirmed. When the type of institution was taken into account no significant association was discovered between the numbers of children in the living units and the scale scores.

## Hypothesis V

All of the units we studied had staff *assigned* to them in reasonable numbers by today's standards for children's units. The unit with fewest staff, a voluntary home, had a ratio of 1 staff to 9 children. As we had predicted, there was no relationship between assigned staff ratios and scores on the revised Child Management Scale. Obviously there are limits below which staffing cannot be allowed to fall if child-oriented management practices are to be maintained at a meaningful level. On the other hand, the provision of many staff is no guarantee that institutionally-oriented practices will not occur. Thus a hospital with staff assigned to the ward producing a ratio of 1 to 3·42 children had a scale score of 45 compared to 37 points for a hospital ward with an assigned staff ratio of 1 to 8·15.

## Hypothesis VI

Staff in the different institutions we surveyed were used differently, however, and when we calculated *effective* staff ratios for different periods of the day we found that child-oriented units had most staff on duty at 'peak' periods of the daily routine when they were most needed. In institutionally-oriented units this did not happen and there were no differences in their staffing when peak and slack periods were compared.

## Hypothesis VII

We also found, as we predicted, that child-oriented units enjoyed greater continuity of staffing than institutionally-oriented units. This was not simply because of high staff turnover in the hospitals in the accepted sense of the term, but resulted in part from the demands of nurse training courses which required students to move from ward to ward. We estimated that in some mental subnormality hospitals, immature and handicapped children might be required to adjust to as many as 100 different adults or more in the course of a single year. In fairness we should point out that our study was not designed to collect data on staff turnover, and this finding must be regarded as rather more tentative than most of the others.

## Hypothesis VIII

According to this hypothesis we predicted that the activities of heads of units would be related to the patterns of care in their units. We found that the heads of child-oriented units spent a significantly greater proportion of their time in activities which necessarily involved them with the children—Social, Physical and Supervisory Child Care—while the heads of institutionally-oriented units spent significantly more of their time in tasks which did not necessarily involve children—Domestic and Administrative activities.

## Hypothesis IX

Not only did unit heads in child-oriented units organize their time differently, they also managed to interact more frequently and more warmly with the children in the way we predicted, whatever else they were doing at the time, than the heads of institutionally-oriented units. They spoke to the children one-and-a-half times as often, were twice as likely to *accept* and three times less likely to *reject* the children than the heads of institutionally-oriented units. When they were engaged in Domestic or Administrative activities, the heads of child-oriented units tended to undertake them in the presence of children, whereas the heads of institutionally-oriented units did so in isolation from the children. To some extent the same patterns emerged when these variables were examined within institutional types.

## Hypothesis X

We expected there to be a more specialized division of labour in institutionally-oriented units, with tasks being allocated to staff along status lines, whereas child-oriented units would be characterized by greater role diffusion, with members of both senior and junior grades engaged in similar activities. Indeed, this was the case. There were few major differences between the activities of junior staff in different types of establishment, but in child-oriented units the pattern of activities for junior staff more closely resembled that for the heads of their units.

## Hypothesis XI

Although junior staff were required to do much the same tasks in different establishments, they carried them out very differently. We expected junior staff in child-oriented units to interact with the children more frequently and more warmly than their counterparts in institutionally-oriented units, in much the same way as their seniors had done. This expectation was confirmed, with junior staff in hostels talking to children to a significantly greater degree, and *rejecting* children significantly less than junior staff in hospitals.

The findings in relation to the last four hypotheses strongly suggest that the role of the head of the unit and the way she performs it is extremely important in establishing the pattern of care for her unit. We therefore turned our attention to factors which might influence the role of the head of the unit, and her performance of it, and thus in turn influence the patterns of care. We looked at her autonomy and responsibility within the organization in which she worked and at her training.

## Hypothesis XII

We found that there were marked differences between the hostels and the hospitals in the amount of responsibility delegated to unit heads. In neither case were unit heads fully responsible for policy matters in relation to children, but in all other respects the heads of hostels had much more responsibility as measured by our Responsibility Index than heads of wards. They were also subject to less frequent inspection. Since hostel heads were also the ones who spent most time on the Social, Physical and Supervisory care of the children, our hypothesis that the more responsibility given to unit heads the more they will be directly involved with the children was provisionally confirmed. Although the differences in degrees of responsibility among hostels on the one hand and among hospitals on the other were too small to demonstrate any relationship between these variables within institution types, the respective scores for the voluntary homes were all in the predicted direction.

## Hypothesis XIII

When we examined the training of the head of the unit we found considerable support for our hypothesis that high rates of inter-action with the children are associated with training in child care, whereas low rates of interaction were associated with a nursing training. What was so striking about our findings here was that there was overlap between institutions of different types in respect of the training of unit heads. In spite of very small numbers there were statistically significant associations between the training of hostel heads and their role activities, their rates of interaction with the children and also with the revised Child Management

Scale scores of their units. In all cases these findings were in the predicted directions. Moreover the same pattern was found in the voluntary homes where there were units with differently trained heads, and staff training therefore helps to explain some of the wide variations among these units on several variables.

Although the design for our survey did not permit us to test for any possible effects on the children of different patterns of care, we did collect some data in this area. In the field studies we had found that children in hostels were more skilled at feeding and in speech than otherwise comparable children in hospitals. In the survey, it was possible to compare groups of children of similar diagnosis, physical handicaps, age and intelligence in different types of institutions. Those in child-oriented units were significantly more advanced in speech and feeding than those in institutionally-oriented units. We could not, of course, rule out the possibility that such differences resulted from selective factors. Nevertheless, we think it more likely that the greater frequency of talking by staff, more of whom were available at peak times when the children were in the units, and the fact that staff ate with children, thus providing an adult model for them to follow, will account for the higher levels of skill on the part of children in child-oriented units.

## Implications of the studies

The conclusions of a study such as this, in which the hypotheses have been many and the fieldwork limited, must necessarily be tentative. It should be emphasized that the institutions we studied were not selected for their representativeness, and we have no wish to generalize beyond the level that our data permit. At the same time fieldwork in more than 100 living units in twenty-six institutions, which involved many hundreds of hours of observation and interviewing, seems to provide a reasonably firm base from which to discuss some of the issues at stake in the provision of residential services, particularly those for the subnormal.

### Are child-oriented management practices desirable?

This is obviously a political or moral question and not a scientific one. It is none the less a question which has to be answered. In developing our concepts of child-oriented management practices and institutionally-oriented management practices we have been guided as far as possible by the scientific literature on residential institutions. In our attempt to measure management practices

198

operationally we have consciously tried to avoid value judgments, and find objective indices which could be reliably assessed by other observers. But the very terms in the literature, and which we have taken over—rigidity, depersonalization, 'block treatment' and social distance—have an inescapable emotional tone, and no doubt we have not been entirely successful in eliminating a value element from our measures. The reader may judge that for himself.

It is also important to note that the revised Child Management Scale measures only those aspects of daily management included as items in the list in Table 8.1. There are many other matters—for example, the ease of visiting by relatives and the frequency of its occurrence, or the provision of community activities—which are relevant to an assessment of residential care and which are not included in the scale. Nonetheless we believe the scale measures, in a reliable way, many of the most important characteristics of institutional care for children.

Having tried to avoid value judgments in the conduct of our studies, and as far as we could in the writing of this report, we wish to state explicitly our belief that child-oriented management practices are 'better' for children, and therefore more desirable, than institutionally-oriented practices. This is a normative judgment, and one which we do not regard as dependent for its validity on the claim that upbringing in a child-oriented environment will make children healthier, better able to talk, test higher in intelligence, cease to be subnormal or become better adjusted as adults. Any or all of these consequences may follow in individual cases as valuable additional consequences of child-oriented upbringing. But kindliness and consideration, an environment in which children are respected as persons, treated as individuals, and given variety of experience, seem to us important, in our society and at this time, whether or not they benefit children in measurable terms. We would prefer that we ourselves or our children might be brought up in the hostel or the voluntary home described in Chapter 7 rather than in the hospital ward. And we think that inasmuch as other children are treated in a manner which is impersonal and institutional, not only do they suffer but the community also loses something of its respect for human dignity and human happiness. Of course, if it could be shown that child-oriented practices had consequences which were actually harmful one would have to think again—to try to balance the losses and gains to be had from adopting other policies. There is no suggestion that this is a real issue. The evidence is rather that there are likely to be long-term benefits from what we think of as 'good' treatment, as well as immediate rewards. But much further research is required before the effects of different forms of institutional upbringing can be adequately assessed.

We assume that there would be general agreement in this country today that child-oriented practices were the more desirable, that they should be maintained where they exist and that they should be striven for where they do not. Certainly the national Press publicity given to alleged incidents in mental hospitals and to the problems of caring for the subnormal (*News of the World,* 20 August 1967; *Guardian,* 28 March and 11 December 1968, 7 January and 25 September 1969; *Observer,* 21 and 28 September; *Sunday Times,* 28 September 1969) suggests that this is the case. Following the Report of the Ely Hospital Inquiry (1969), set up to investigate the allegations of ill treatment of patients and other irregularities at Ely Hospital, Cardiff, the Minister of Health established a working party to consider the needs of the services for the subnormal. The working party has considered many possibilities for the alleviation of problems in subnormality hospitals, as well as longer-term reforms. But as Wing and Brown (1970) have shown, reform in hospitals for the mentally ill has a natural history and efforts have to be constantly kept up. It is to be expected that the reform of the mental deficiency services will be subject to similar pressures, and that short-term expedients, while necessary, will not be sufficient to achieve and maintain child-oriented patterns of care. It therefore seems worthwhile to discuss the implications of some of our findings in this context.

## Size of institutions and living units

Our evidence did not support the view that all large establishments are necessarily 'institutional' in character, or that large living units with forty or more children in them are necessarily impersonal. The type of institution, and its organizational structure, was much more important than size in influencing the patterns of care as measured by our scale. Large children's homes were able to maintain child-oriented patterns of care, as were hostels with comparatively large living units. Even small hospitals, and hospitals with small living units, on the other hand, had institutional patterns of care. But size is a complex issue, and there is no reason to suppose that it should affect the particular items included on our scale.

The arguments against large institutions are concerned with other matters. Briefly, they are that a large institution is inevitably more cut off from the general community than a small one, and draws its members from a much wider geographical area. As a result, it is difficult for parents to visit and maintain contact with their children, which later makes for problems in the eventual rehabilitation of patients. It is probable, too, that there are greater problems in recruiting and holding staff for the large and isolated establishment. These arguments have been spelt out more fully elsewhere (Tizard, 1964, 1970). It may also be the case that the larger the institution, the more difficult it is to allow a household-type organization for the living units, and the more likely that the organization will be centralized. The history of mental institutions suggests that the larger the institutions have become, the harder it has been to eschew the obvious attractions of centralization and to maintain an appropriate balance with the social environment 'outside'.

The arguments against large living units were well expressed by the Curtis Committee a quarter of a century ago. In the case of younger, handicapped and immature children, it is likely that only small groups of others can be tolerated and understood. The larger is the living unit, the greater the volume of noise, the more strangers, and the more inevitable confusion. Even for adults, large living units are undesirable because they are uncomfortable and inhuman places in which to live.

For all these reasons, our personal preference is for establishments and for living units which are small in size. But simply reducing the size of establishments and living units, as our data show, does nothing *in itself* to change the daily pattern of care, and provides no guarantee that they will become more child-oriented, without other action being taken.

*Staffing*

The reason usually given for inadequacies in child care in institutions for the handicapped is shortage of staff. In many institutions this is a valid reason. But it is not sufficient. Ely hospital was doubtless understaffed, but the recommendations of the Ely Hospital Inquiry (1969) to double the staffing establishment then specified for the children's villas (para. 522) would provide no guarantee of establishing child-oriented patterns of care in those villas—though it might have gone a long way to alleviate other problems. Even well-staffed units can be run in an institutionally-oriented manner if the staff are not properly organized and if they do not receive the right kind of training. Attention needs to be paid to the difficult organizational problem of ensuring that most staff are on duty at the times when they are most needed, without overburdening staff with unduly long and inconvenient hours of work. It is also important to ensure as much stability in the staffing of units as possible. There are no simple solutions,

201

P

and the problem should not be oversimplified to just a question of numbers. One thing in the hospital setting which might be reconsidered, however, is the necessity for moving student nurses from one ward to another as part of their training. Since the patterns of care do not markedly differ from one ward to another at present, there seems little to be gained educationally from this exercise.

## The responsibilities and training of staff

The findings of the present studies point overwhelmingly to the importance of the role of the head of the living unit in setting the patterns for the ward or hostel. If these findings can be taken at their face value, they suggest that relieving the unit head of responsibility for everything but child care is *not* a good way of ensuring that she spends most of her time on this activity. On the contrary, unit heads who have more rather than less responsibility, and who are inspected by superiors less frequently, are, according to this evidence, the ones who promoted the most active child-oriented practices of upbringing. We suspect, although we did not examine the matter directly, that in such units the senior staff feel a deeper sense of responsibility towards the children and a deeper sense of commitment to the unit as a whole.

There seems to be everything to be said for attempting to involve staff more directly with the children. In the light of these findings, it seems a pity that the Ely Hospital Inquiry concluded, on quite different grounds, that 'nurses must not be permitted to take meals on the ward', and that 'special accommodation should be provided where those who bring their own food in the hospital can eat' (para. 538). It seems to us that the fact that hostel and voluntary home staff not only ate in the units, but *ate with the children,* might be responsible for the greater skills of self-feeding of the children in their units: staff eating with the children certainly contributed towards the homely atmosphere of their units.

The consistency of the relationship between staff activities and the patterns of child management as between hostels and hospitals in our study was one of the most persistent features of our research. Nevertheless, there were differences within the hostels on some variables (and also in the voluntary homes) which could be directly related to the training of staff. Although we did not examine the content of training syllabuses, our data provide quantitative support to those who argue that nurse training, as at present organized, is an unsatisfactory preparation for work in the long-term care of the handicapped. There are certainly grounds for re-examining the nature and content of nurse training for the care of the subnormal, and there are courses available in child care which might well serve as suitable models in any reconstruction.

## Future research

From the point of view of the sociology of residential organizations, we have found the problems of conceptualizing the relevant dimensions for analysis—and translating them into operational terms—the most difficult part of the study. We are well aware that all the difficulties have by no means been surmounted. None the less, we feel a beginning has been made towards the systematic comparative analysis of the structure and function of these hybrid establishments.

It is, of course, customary to conclude monographs of this kind with a plea for more research, and we do so here. We have tried to present our material in such a way that the work can be replicated, and we have tried to give sufficient detail about methods in the text and in the Appendices to facilitate this. There is clearly a need for larger-scale validation studies, using survey techniques. But there are limits to the problems that can be encompassed by the survey, and the real need is for experiment in which changes in the patterns of care may be effected—and evaluated. The opportunities for experiment are there if we will grasp them. And social experiment may bring rewards no less great than those which have come from experiment in the physical and biological sciences.

Further research which extends and tests the work outlined in this monograph is indeed already under way. Working from the Department of Child Development of the University of London Institute of Education, Kushlick and his colleagues, in conjunction with the Wessex Regional Hospital Board and selected Local Authorities, are carrying out a series of experimental studies of different types of residential care for mentally retarded children. The effects upon the children and their families, and the social and organizational problems which arise out of contrasting patterns of care, are being studied over time, as are costs and the impact of the newly instituted forms of service upon other health, education and welfare services (Kushlick, 1968).

Also in the Department of Child Development of the Institute of Education Barbara Tizard and colleagues have been looking at factors affecting the upbringing of normal pre-school children in residential care. This research is concerned with the inter-relationships between (1) aspects of the organizational structure of the different residential nurseries and (2) the patterns of staff-child interaction and (3) the development of young children in residential care (Tizard, 1970, 1971).

Working from the Department of Sociology and Social Administration in the University of Southampton, King and his colleagues are using a similar research strategy to measure differences in the régimes in a number of prisons, and to study the effects of these upon the prisoners who experience them.

The range of these additional studies makes us confident that the method of approach developed in the Child Welfare Project is both useful and flexible.

# Appendices

# I The revised Child Management Scale

The revised Child Management Scale consisted of thirty items which are reproduced below. Scoring categories and the data sources are given for each item. A score of 0 indicates child-orientation; a score of 2 indicates institutional-orientation; a score of 1 indicates a mixed pattern. Items marked (AC) were asked only of specified ambulant children randomly selected from within each unit. Items marked * were included in the original Inmate Management Scale (King and Raynes, 1968a).

The data were collected from interviews and observations. The main instruments were the Child Management Interview (Form B1), and the Observation Check List (Form B2). Many items were collected from both these sources. One item (No. 17) was based on data collected using the Children's Questionnaire (Form A2). These forms are reproduced in Appendices II and III. Some of the items recorded on the Observation Check List were in turn based on information recorded during the Long Day (Staff Activities) Observations (Form C2), which is reproduced in Appendix III.

## Rigidity of Routine

Management practices are institutionally-oriented when they are inflexible from one day to the next, and from one inmate to another; individuals in different situations are treated as though they were in the same situation, and changes in circumstances are not taken into account. Management practices are child-oriented when they are flexible, being adapted to take into account individual differences among the children or different circumstances.

| *Items* | *Data Source* |
|---|---|
| 1. (AC)* Do the children aged 5 years and over get up at the same time at weekends as they do during the week?<br>0 Different times for all on 2 days<br>1 Different for some, or on 1 day only<br>2 Same time | B1 (3) |

| *Items* | | *Data Source* |
|---|---|---|
| 2. (AC)* | Do the children aged 5 years and over go to bed at the same time at weekends as they do during the week? | B1 (25) |
| | 0 Different times for all on 2 days | |
| | 1 Different for some, or on 1 day only | |
| | 2 Same time | |
| 3. (AC)* | Do they use the yard or garden at set times? | B1 (37) |
| | 0 No, whenever they like | B2 (24) |
| | 1 Under various conditions | |
| | 2 Yes, set times only | |
| 4. (AC)* | Do they use their bedrooms at set times? | B1 (33) |
| | 0 No, whenever they like | |
| | 1 Under various conditions | |
| | 2 Yes, set times only | |
| 5. | Are there set times when visitors can come to the unit? | B1 (44) |
| | 0 Any time (except during specified times) | |
| | 1 Any day, but set times | |
| | 2 Certain days only | |
| 6. | Which children are routinely toileted at night? | B1 (26) |
| | 0 None/some only once | |
| | 1 Some more than once | |
| | 2 All once or more | |

### 'Block Treatment'

Child management practices are institutionally-oriented if the children are regimented – that is, all dealt with as a group – before, during or after any specific activity. These practices involve queueing and waiting around, with large groups of other children and with no mode of occupation during the waiting period. Management practices may be described as child-oriented where the organization of activity is such that residents are allowed to participate or not as they please, and where they are allowed to do things at their own pace.

| *Items* | | *Data Source* |
|---|---|---|
| 7. (AC) | After getting dressed, do the children wait around doing nothing? | B1 (5) |
| | | B2 (1) |
| | 0 No, they are occupied | |
| | 1 Some wait doing nothing | |
| | 2 Everybody waits doing nothing | |
| 8. (AC)* | Do they wait in line before coming in for breakfast? | B1 (5) |
| | | B2 (2) |
| | 0 None wait | |
| | 1 Some wait | |
| | 2 All wait | |

| *Items* | | *Data Source* |
|---|---|---|
| 9. (AC)* | Do they wait together as a group before bathing? | B1 (22) B2 (17) |

9. (AC)* Do they wait together as a group before bathing?
B1 (22)
B2 (17)
0 None wait, all occupied elsewhere
1 Some wait, or mixed pattern
2 All wait

10. (AC)* Do they wait together as a group after bathing?
B1 (23)
B2 (18)
0 None wait, return individually
1 Some wait, or mixed pattern
2 All wait

11. (AC) How do they return from the toilet?
B1 (4, 8, 13, 16, 19)
B2 (14)
0 Individually
1 In groups, or mixed pattern
2 All together

12. (AC) Do they sit waiting at tables before the meal is served? (tea or evening meal)
B2 (3, 4, 5, 6)
0 Less than 5 minutes (mean day 1 and day 2)
1 6–10 minutes
2 More than 10 minutes

13. (AC)* Do they sit waiting at tables after the meal is finished and before next activity? (tea or evening meal)
B2 (7, 8, 9)
0 Less than 7 minutes (mean day 1 and day 2)
1 8–14 minutes
2 15 or more minutes

14. (AC) How are the children organized when they go on walks?
B1 (39)
B2 (23)
0 Taken a few at a time
1 All at once, but in separate groups
2 In 'crocodiles' or similar

## Depersonalization

Child management practices may be seen as institutionally-oriented when there are no opportunities for residents to have personal possessions or personal privacy. Depersonalization is also shown where there is an absence of opportunities for self-expression, or of situations in which initiative on the part of the child may be shown. Where there are opportunities for residents to show initiative, to have personal possessions, to be alone if they so desire, the child management practices may be described as child-oriented.

*Items*                                                    *Data Source*
15.       What is done with the children's private         B1 (28)
          clothing?                                        B2 (26)
          0 Kept and used by children
          1 Used only on visits, special occasions
          2 Not used or not allowed

| *Items* | | *Data Source* |
|---|---|---|
| 16. | What is done with the children's private toys? | B1 (29) |
| | | B2 (27) |

0 Kept and used by children
1 Kept for a time, but become communal
2 Not used or not allowed

17.* How many of the children possess *all* of the   A2 (23)
following articles of clothing: shirt or blouse,
trousers or skirt, dress or jacket, jumper,
topcoat, shoes, dressing gown, slippers?
0 67 – 100%
1 34 – 66%
2 0 – 33%

18.* Whereabouts do they keep their daily clothes?   B1 (30)
  B2 (28)

0 In private provision
1 In shared provision, supplied weekly
2 In communal provision, supplied daily

19.* How many children have toys or books of   B1 (32)
their own?
0 67 – 100%
1 34 – 66%
2 0 – 33%

20. Do they have pictures, pin-ups, photos in   B2 (30)
rooms?
0 Yes, in all rooms
1 In some rooms
2 No

21. How much time do they have for playing?   B2 (25)
0 At least $\frac{1}{2}$ hour each day of observation
1 At least $\frac{1}{4}$ hour each day of observation
2 Less than this

22. How are children's birthdays celebrated?   B1 (47)
0 Individual presents or parties
1 Mixed pattern
2 Joint parties or no recognition

23. How are tables laid for meals? (tea or evening   B2 (10)
meal)
0 Tables laid for all children
1 Tables laid for some children
2 Not laid – food and spoon handed out by staff

Note: The term 'private' means clothes or articles provided by parents or
relations. For all other items, ownership is not required: it is
sufficient for children to have sole, permanent use of the articles,
whatever their source, for possession to be established.

## Social Distance

Management practices are institutionally-oriented when there is a sharp separation between the staff and inmate worlds. This may be because separate areas of accommodation are kept for the exclusive use of staff, or because interaction between staff and children is limited to formal, and functionally specific, activities. Child orientation involves the reduction of social distance by the sharing of living space, and allows staff and children to interact in functionally diffuse and informal situations.

| *Items* | | *Data Source* |
|---|---|---|
| 24. (AC)* | Do the children have any access to the kitchen? | B1 (34) |
| | | B2 (20) |
| | 0  67 – 100% | |
| | 1  34 – 66% | |
| | 2  0 – 33% | |
| 25. (AC)* | Do the children have any access to other areas? | B1 (35, 36) |
| | | B2 (21) |
| | 0  Yes, no restrictions | |
| | 1  To some areas | |
| | 2  No, doors are kept locked | |
| 26. | How do staff assist children at toilet times? | B2 (13) |
| | 0  One staff member for each child | |
| | 1  Mixed pattern | |
| | 2  'Conveyor-belt' system | |
| | ('Conveyor-belt' system means that one child passes through the hands of two or more members of staff during this routine.) | |
| 27.* | How do staff assist children at bath times? | B2 (19) |
| | 0  One staff member for each child | |
| | 1  Mixed pattern | |
| | 2  'Conveyor-belt' system | |
| 28.* | Do staff on duty eat with the children? (tea or evening meal) | B2 (11) |
| | 0  All staff (at least sometimes) | |
| | 1  Some staff, or sit but don't eat | |
| | 2  Stand, serve and supervise only | |
| 29. | Do staff on duty sit and watch TV with children? | B1 (40) |
| | | B2 (22) |
| | 0  Someone usually does | |
| | 1  Someone sometimes does | |
| | 2  Sporadic supervision only | |
| 30. (AC) | How many children have been on outings with staff in last 3 months? | B1 (42) |
| | 0  67 – 100% | |
| | 1  34 – 66% | |
| | 2  0 – 33% | |

211

Both the original Inmate Management Scale and the revised Child Management Scale were developed in the same way. In our early studies, a pool of items was devised which related to comparable areas of child management practice in homes for the deprived as well as institutions for the handicapped. In our later studies, we were able to expand the pool of items because our attention was limited to establishments for the subnormal, where a greater number of practices might be compared.

Most items were derived from data collected using the Child Management Interview (Form B1) and the Observation Check list (Form B2). Both instruments were found to be reliable in use (see Appendix II).

The two sociologists (R. D. K. and N. V. R.) rated each item on a three-point scale, 0, 1 or 2, and any item which could not be unambiguously scored in this way was discarded. Each unit in the study was then scored independently by the two raters, with a level of agreement between them of 94·6 per cent. An agreed rating was made following discussion in those cases where discrepancies existed. After any items which appeared to be dependent on age, handicap or cultural factors were eliminated, a pool of forty-five items was left for analysis.

Once all the items were scored, a simple item analysis was carried out following the procedures suggested by Maxwell (1961). First, the items were examined for their discriminating power, by inspecting the frequency of the score of 0. Maxwell recommends that any item for which more than 80 per cent or less than 20 per cent of the responses are favourable should be discarded because of failure to discriminate. Second, the items were inspected for their linearity. This was done by arranging the units into four groups from the lowest to the highest scorers when all the items were added together. The distribution of scores for each item were then compared with the distribution of scores for all items. Maxwell recommends that any items which do not show a linear distribution should also be excluded.

All except five of the scale items listed above were shown to be efficient discriminators, and also had linear distributions. They were included in the scale because they met both the criteria suggested by Maxwell. Four items (numbers 3, 8, 10 and 28) were found to be satisfactory in terms of discrimination and linearity when the original scale was developed in the field studies, but failed one or both these tests on the data from the survey. These items were included in the revised scale simply because they had constituted part of the original scale. In any case, they very nearly met the criteria for inclusion.

Maxwell suggested that if there was doubt about the inclusion of an item, on the basis of discrimination or linearity, a Chi square test should be applied to the data. All items from the pool which met only one of the criteria were therefore subjected to a Chi square test, using the Yates correction. Only one of the items tested in this way was statistically significant, and this was included in the scale as item 12.

Of the remaining fifteen items, seven met only one of Maxwell's criteria and were not statistically significant when a Chi square test was performed:

31. How many children use the yard or gardens?

32. Is tea served at the same time at weekends?

33. Have children had friends in, or themselves been out to tea or play, in the last three months?

34. How often do they go on walks?

35. How many go to clubs or activities outside?

36. How many have been shopping with staff in the last three months?

37. Do staff talk to the children at teatime?

These items were therefore eliminated. A further six items met none of the criteria, and were eliminated. These were:

38. Which children are toileted at routine sessions?

39. Is there a set time for bathing?

40. How are ambulant children taken to the toilet?

41. Are doors to the unit kept locked?

42. How is the lifting of children at night organized?

43. How many children go out on walks with staff?

Two items were seen to be dependent on other items already included in the scale, and were excluded on that ground:

44. Where do children keep their toys or books?

45. Was the children's clothing marked in any way?

The original Inmate Management Scale was developed in 4 institutions containing 79 separate living units. Altogether, it has been applied in 88 living units 82 of which were reported on in Part II of this monograph. That scale contained 16 items. Two of these items, 'How many have toys of their own?' and 'How many have books of any kind of their own?' which were appropriately asked separately when we were comparing institutions for the deprived as well as for the subnormal, were collapsed to form the present item 19 when we confined our attention to institutions for the subnormal. The revised Child Management Scale was developed and applied in 1 living unit in each of 16 institutions for the subnormal, after piloting in 4 other institutions. It contains the 15 items of the original scale, and 15 new items. The correlation between the old items and the new items, for the 16 institutions studied in the survey, was $r = 0.92$.

# II   Questionnaires, interviews and recording schedules

## Form A1: Children's Questionnaire

This schedule was completed by the fieldworker from information in the case records for each child.

| | Leave blank Col. 7 | | Leave blank Col. 7 |
|---|---|---|---|
| | | FORM A1<br>CHILDREN'S QUESTIONNAIRE<br><br>STRICTLY CONFIDENTIAL | Office use only<br><br>Estab.<br>Unit<br>Child |

| | Leave blank Col. 7 | | Leave blank Col. 7 |
|---|---|---|---|
| | | 5 + years | 7 |
| 1. Male | 0 | 10 + „ | 8 |
| Female | 1 | No information | X |
| 2. Date of birth | 8 | 4. Number of other wards | |
| 0 – 1 | 0 | child has been on | 10 |
| 2 – 4 | 1 | 5. Date of admission to | |
| 5 –10 | 2 | present ward | 12 |
| 11–14 | 3 | 6. Mongol | 0 |
| 15+ | 4 | Non-Mongol | 1 |
| No information | X | No information | X |
| 3. Date of current admission | | 7. Latest IQ assessment | |
| | 9 | Score | |
| 0 – 2 months | 0 | Test | |
| 3 – 5 „ | 1 | Date | |
| 6 –11 „ | 2 | 8. Latest M.A. | |
| 1 year | 3 | M.A. | |
| 2 years | 4 | Test | |
| 3 „ | 5 | Date | |
| 4 „ | 6 | | |

214

| 9. Estimate | | | 10.Final assessment | | 13 |
|---|---|---|---|---|---|
| Idiot | 0·20 | | Idiot | 0 –20 | 0 |
| Low imbecile | 21–30 | | Low imbecile | 21–30 | 1 |
| Medium imbecile | 31–40 | | Medium imbecile | 31–40 | 2 |
| High imbecile | 41–50 | | High imbecile | 41–50 | 3 |
| Feeble-minded | 51+ | | Feeble-minded | 51+ | 4 |
| No information | | | No information | | X |
| Source | | | | | |

## Form A2: Children's Questionnaire

This schedule was completed, after the fieldwork was finished, by the head of the unit. One questionnaire was completed for each child, and each unit head was given a folder containing all the questionnaires, together with a set of notes of guidance. These notes are given at the end of the schedule. The fieldworker in each establishment went through one specimen form with the head of the unit, to make sure there were no ambiguities. The completed schedules were returned by post to the research unit in a pre-paid envelope which was also left with the head of the unit. All the unit heads returned satisfactorily completed schedules on each of their children.

| FORM A2<br>CHILDREN'S QUESTIONNAIRE<br><br>STRICTLY CONFIDENTIAL | Office use only<br><br>Estab.<br>Unit<br>Child |
|---|---|

1. Please state
   Name of child
   Name of establishment
   Name or number of unit

| *Section 1* | *Leave blank Col.* | | *Leave blank Col.* |
|---|---|---|---|
| 2. Does child feed self? (*see notes) | | 4. Is child able to communicate by speech? (*see notes) | |
| Yes, with knife and fork | 0 | Yes, sentences and normal | 0 |
| Yes, with spoon | 1 | Yes, odd words only | 1 |
| Needs help | 2 | No recognizable speech | 2 |
| Has to be fed | 3 | | X |
| | X | 5. Does child have any difficulty with sight? (*see notes) | |
| 3. Does child dress self? (*see notes) | | | |
| Yes, unaided | 0 | Yes, blind or almost blind | 0 |
| Yes, apart from buttons, etc. | 1 | Yes, has poor sight | 1 |
| No, needs more help | 2 | No, normal sight | 2 |
| No, has to be dressed | 3 | | X |
| | X | | |

**215**

6. Does child have any difficulty with hearing? (*see notes)

| | |
|---|---|
| Yes, deaf or almost deaf | 0 |
| Yes, poor hearing | 1 |
| No, normal hearing | 2 |
| | X |

7. Does this child have fits or turns? (*see notes)

| | |
|---|---|
| Yes | 1 |
| No | 2 |
| | X |

8. Does child wet self during day?

| | |
|---|---|
| At least once a day | 0 |
| At least once a week | 1 |
| At least once a month | 2 |
| Rarely or never | 3 |
| | X |

9. Does child wet self at night?

| | |
|---|---|
| At least once a night | 0 |
| At least once a week | 1 |
| At least once a month | 2 |
| Rarely or never | 3 |
| | X |

10. Does child soil self during day?

| | |
|---|---|
| At least once a day | 0 |
| At least once a week | 1 |
| At least once a month | 2 |
| Rarely or never | 3 |
| | X |

11. Does child soil self at night?

| | |
|---|---|
| At least once a night | 0 |
| At least once a week | 1 |
| At least once a month | 2 |
| Rarely or never | 3 |
| | X |

12. Is child able to walk or move about by self?

| | |
|---|---|
| Yes, walks unaided | 0 |
| Yes, shuffles on bottom | 1 |
| Yes, in self-propelled wheel-chair | 2 |
| No, needs some assistance | 3 |
| No, has to be moved or carried | 4 |
| | X |

## Section 2

Below are a series of descriptions of behaviour and problems which are shown by some children. If the child, AS HE IS NOW, does NOT show the behaviour, put a cross in the box in column 1. If the child *definitely* shows the behaviour, put a cross in the box in column 3. If the child behaves *somewhat* according to the statement, put a cross in the box in column 2 (* see notes).

| | 1 Does not apply | 2 Somewhat applies | 3 Certainly applies |
|---|---|---|---|
| 13. Hits out or attacks others | ☐ | ☐ | ☐ |
| 14. Extremely overactive. Does not sit down a minute. Paces up and down restlessly | ☐ | ☐ | ☐ |
| 15. Constantly seeking attention – will not leave adults | ☐ | ☐ | ☐ |
| 16. Tears up papers, clothing or damages furniture | ☐ | ☐ | ☐ |
| 17. Continually injuring himself physically, e.g. head banging, picking sores, beating eyes | ☐ | ☐ | ☐ |
| 18. Absconds, attempts to abscond, e.g. often missing or would be if not closely watched | ☐ | ☐ | ☐ |
| 19. Has temper tantrums, or screaming fits | ☐ | ☐ | ☐ |
| 20. Is withdrawn or solitary | ☐ | ☐ | ☐ |

216

*Section 3*

| | | Leave blank Col. |
|---|---|---|

**21.** Has any arrangement been made for this child to be visited by an adult other than his parents (e.g. friends from the hospital)?

Yes ☐    0
No ☐    1
    X

**22.** How often has the child been visited by people from outside the establishment?

| | Relatives | Others | |
|---|---|---|---|
| Weekly | ☐ | ☐ | 0 |
| Fortnightly | ☐ | ☐ | 1 |
| Monthly | ☐ | ☐ | 2 |
| Less often | ☐ | ☐ | 3 |
| Not at all | ☐ | ☐ | 4 |
| | | | X |

**23.** Below are a list of items. For each time, put an X in column 1 if the child possesses it. Put an X in column 2 if he does not (*see notes).

| | Col. 1 | Col. 2 |
|---|---|---|
| Underwear | ☐ | ☐ |
| Shirt or blouse | ☐ | ☐ |
| Trousers or skirt | ☐ | ☐ |
| Dress, suit or jacket | ☐ | ☐ |
| Jumper or cardigan | ☐ | ☐ |
| Top coat | ☐ | ☐ |
| Pair of shoes | ☐ | ☐ |
| Pyjamas | ☐ | ☐ |
| Dressing gown | ☐ | ☐ |
| Slippers or houseshoes | ☐ | ☐ |

THANK YOU VERY MUCH FOR YOUR HELP

---

### NOTES OF GUIDANCE

This questionnaire is divided into THREE sections. Please ensure that you have marked one box for every question – no question should be completely blank when you have finished. The following notes should help you in deciding your answers.

Section 1

2. Answer as the child actually *does* feed now, not how he might or could if there were more time.
3. Answer how the child actually *does* dress now, not how he might or could if there were more time.
4. 'Yes, sentences and normal' here would include a number of children with speech defects, so long as they can communicate in understandable sentences of a simple kind.
5. With spectacles, if normally worn. 'Poor sight' would include children who have to move closer to the TV or peer closely at books before they can see satisfactorily.
6. With hearing aid, if normally worn. 'Poor hearing' would include children who make compensatory movements, e.g. incline the head in order to hear, or who can hear when things are said slowly and clearly.
7. If the child has had no fits since being in your care, and receives no current medication for them, record as 'No', even if there is a history.

Section 2

For these questions, it is important that you record how the child behaves *now* in your unit. If the child is receiving *current* medication, which affects his behaviour, answer according to how he actually behaves now, under medication.

Section 3

23. For this question, it is not necessary that the child should own the items in order to possess them. He can possess them *either* if they are provided for him

**217**

P

privately, *or* if they are provided by your establishment and he has sole and permanent use of them. This would apply, for example, if the child got the same shirt returned to him each time from the laundry. If he got a different shirt each time, he could not be said to possess it.

### Form B1: Child Management Schedule

This interview schedule provided much of the data subsequently used for the scale items listed in Appendix I. An earlier draft of the schedule was used in the field studies, and in all the schedule has been used in more than 100 units for children. The interview is conducted with the head of the unit – ward sister, charge nurse or housemother. Reliability of the interview was assessed in the following way: in six units, the Child Management Interviews were conducted by two interviewers, and the responses recorded by each interviewer on every question were compared. The number of agreed responses were then expressed as a percentage of the total responses. The level of agreement varied from 88·6 to 96·4 per cent, the mean level being 94·2 per cent. For the sake of brevity, a number of questions which did not yield possible scale items and which were not necessary to maintain the flow of the interview have been omitted, and the space allowed for recording has been reduced.

---

FORM B1
CHILD MANAGEMENT SCHEDULE

STRICTLY CONFIDENTIAL

Office use only

Estab.
Unit
Date

---

*I want to talk to you about the children in your ward, especially the following ambulant children. First, I want to go through their daily activities with you as they happened YESTERDAY, and afterwards to discuss some other aspects of their lives. Before we begin, I should like to emphasize that all your replies will be treated in the strictest confidence.*

---

1. Can I first check the numbers of children who are:
   (a) Ambulant
   (b) Non-ambulant
   (c) Under 5
   (d) Over 5 < 16
   (e) 16 and over

2. What time did the ambulant children over 5 years get up yesterday?
   first child
   last child

3. Do they always get up at this time?

| | |
|---|---|
| All yes | 2 |
| Yes, except on specified days | 1 |
| All no | 0 |
| Other | X |

4. What happened between waking and getting dressed?

| | |
|---|---|
| Toileted/washed | 2 |
| Left in beds | 1 |
| Play | 0 |

*Probe:* Who supervises?
How taken and return?
How many included?

5. What happened between
   dressing and breakfast?
   Nothing                                    2
   Help with breakfast                        1
   Playing                                    0
   *Probe:* Line up at breakfast?

6. What time was breakfast?
   began
   ended

7. Is it always at that time?
   Always                                     2
   Different on specified days                1
   Different weekends                         0

8. What did they do after
   breakfast?
   Toileted/washed                            2
   Help clear away                            1
   Play                                       0
   Other                                      X
   *Probe:* Who supervises?
           How taken and
           return?
           How many involved?

9. How many went to
   morning school (etc.)?
   Industrial training
   Occupational therapy
   School/training centre
   Other
   *Probe:* Time left?
           Who took them?

10. Did they return for
    midday meal?
    Industrial training
    Occupational therapy
    School/training centre
    Other
    *Probe:* Time return?
            Who brought them?

11. What time was lunch?
    began
    ended

12. Is it always that time?
    Always                                    2
    Different on specified days               1
    Different weekends                        0

13. What happened after
    lunch?
    Toileted/washed                           2
    Help clear away                           1
    Play                                      0
    Other                                     X

*Probe:* Who supervises?
        How taken and return?
        How many involved?

14. How many went to after-
    noon school (etc.)?
    Industrial training
    Occupational therapy
    School/training centre
    Other
    *Probe:* Time left?
            Who took them?

15. What time did they return?
    Industrial training
    Occupational therapy
    School/training centre
    Other
    *Probe:* Who brought them?

16. What happened after
    return?
    Toileted/washed                           2
    Help prepare tea                          1
    Play                                      0
    Other                                     X
    *Probe:* Who supervises?
            How taken and
            return?
            How many involved?

17. What time was tea?
    began
    ended

18. Is it always at that time?
    Always                                    2
    Different on specified days               1
    Different weekends                        0

19. What happened after tea?
    Toileted/washed                           2
    Help clear tables                         1
    Play                                      0
    Other                                     X
    *Probe:* Who supervises?
            How taken and
            return?
            How many involved?

20. Were any bathed
    yesterday?
    How many?

21. How often are they
    bathed?
    Daily                                     2
    3 times or more per week                  1
    Weekly                                    0
    Other                                     X

219

22. What do they do immediately before their baths?

| | |
|---|---|
| All wait in group | 2 |
| Some wait in group | 1 |
| All occupied elsewhere | 0 |
| Other | X |

23. What do they do immediately after their baths?

| | |
|---|---|
| All wait in group | 2 |
| Some wait in group | 1 |
| All leave immediately | 0 |
| Other | X |

24. What time did the ambulant children over 5 years go to bed?
    first child
    last child

25. Do they always go to bed at that time?

| | |
|---|---|
| All yes | 2 |
| Yes, except on specified days | 1 |
| All no | 0 |
| Other | X |

26. Which children are lifted for toileting at night?
    changed
    potted
    toileted
    *Probe:* Number of times
           How organized ?

27. So can I now check the routine toilet sessions through the day and night:

| *Session* | *No. of children* |
|---|---|
| ———— | ———— |
| ———— | ———— |
| ———— | ———— |
| ———— | ———— |
| ———— | ———— |
| ———— | ———— |
| ———— | ———— |
| ———— | ———— |

*Now I should like to talk about a number of other aspects relating to the the children:*

28. What is done with the clothes they bring with them?

| | |
|---|---|
| Kept but not used/not allowed | 2 |
| Used visits or special occasions | 1 |
| Used normally | 0 |
| Other | X |

29. What is done with the toys they bring with them?

| | |
|---|---|
| Kept but not used/not allowed | 2 |
| Used but become communal | 1 |
| Used by the children | 0 |
| Other | X |

30. Where do they keep daily clothes?

| | |
|---|---|
| Communal store, daily supplies | 2 |
| Shared provision, weekly supplies | 1 |
| Private provision | 0 |
| Other | X |

31. Are clothes marked in any way?

| | |
|---|---|
| No, or unit mark only | 2 |
| Yes, some items | 1 |
| Yes, all with name or symbol | 0 |

32. How many have toys or books of their own?
    number

33. When may they use bedrooms?

| | |
|---|---|
| Only at bedtimes or to change | 2 |
| Under supervision | 1 |
| Any time | 0 |
| Other | X |

*Probe:* Which children?

34. When may they use kitchen?

| | |
|---|---|
| Not at all | 2 |
| Under supervision | 1 |
| Any time | 0 |
| Other | X |

*Probe:* Which children?

35. What other rooms are there?
_____
_____
_____
_____

36. When may they use the —room? (Repeat as necessary)
Not at all — 2
Under supervision — 1
Any time — 0
Other — X
*Probe:* Which children?

37. When may they use the yard or garden?
Not at all, or at specified times — 2
Under supervision — 1
Any time — 0
Other — X
*Probe:* Which children?

38. How many have been on walks in grounds with staff in last month?
number

39. How are these organized?
Go all together — 2
Go together, but split up — 1
Individually or groups — 0
Other — X

40. Do staff sit and watch TV with children?
No, supervise only — 2
Yes, sometimes — 1
Yes, usually — 0
Other — X

41. How many have been shopping with staff in last month?
number

42. How many have been on outings (seaside, picnic, cinema, etc.) with staff in last three months?
number
place

43. How many go to outside clubs or activities?
number
place

44. When can relatives visit unit?
Certain days only — 2
Any day, but set times — 1
Any time (except during specified activities) — 0
Other — X

45. Have any had friends in to tea or play in last three months?
number

46. Have any been out to friends for tea or play in last 3 months?
number

47. How are birthdays celebrated?
Joint parties/no recognition — 2
Mixed pattern — 1
Individual presents, parties — 0
Other — X

48. How many children have been home for a night or longer during the last 3 months?
number

THANK YOU VERY MUCH FOR YOUR HELP

## Form C1: Timetable for the week

This sheet – one for each day – was used to record the hours of duty for all members of staff working in the unit for the week of the fieldwork. It was completed with the help of the head of the unit.

Estab. ———
Unit ———

| | | 30 11 | 30 10 | 30 9 | 30 8 | 30 7 | 30 6 | 30 5 | 30 4 | 30 3 | 30 2 | 30 1 | 30 12 | 30 11 | 30 10 | 30 9 | 30 8 | 30 7 | 30 6 |
|---|---|---|---|---|---|---|---|---|---|---|---|---|---|---|---|---|---|---|---|

FORM C1
TIMETABLE FOR THIS WEEK

Day
Unit

| Name | Desig-nation | |
|------|--------------|---|
| | | |

## Form C3: Unit Organization Schedule

This schedule was used in an interview with the head of each unit studied. For brevity, the space allowed for recording has been greatly reduced.

---

| FORM C3 | Office use only |
| UNIT ORGANIZATION SCHEDULE | |

STRICTLY CONFIDENTIAL

Estab.
Unit
Date

---

I would like to talk to you about the way your ward/hostel/cottage is organized, and about what it is like to work in a unit like this. Once again, may I assure you that your answers will be treated as confidential.

---

1. First, I would like you to list all the people who work in this unit (for hospital – those who will be working here this week) including domestic staff, night staff and part-time or voluntary helpers.

| Name | Designation | Hours per week | Resident | Non-resident |
|------|-------------|----------------|----------|--------------|
|      |             |                |          |              |
|      |             |                |          |              |

1(a). Is there any one member of staff on call day and night?

Yes    1
No    2

(Be sure to have included all staff, including those off sick, unless you have recorded a replacement for them. If patients help on ward, include these and designate 'ward helper'. If other helpers come in unpaid, include these and designate 'volunteer'.)

2. Whereabouts do the resident staff sleep?

| | Head of unit | Other staff |
|--|--------------|-------------|
| Different building | 0 | 0 |
| Same building, inaccessible | 1 | 1 |
| Same building, accessible | 2 | 2 |
| Non-resident | X | X |

3. Are the children divided up into groups for any activities for any part of the day? (*Probe:* sleeping, eating, school, play, any other activity or reason)

| Activity or purpose | Group | No. of children | Description | Staff | Duration |
|---------------------|-------|-----------------|-------------|-------|----------|
|                     |       |                 |             |       |          |
|                     |       |                 |             |       |          |

Comments on above:

4. Are any members of staff given special responsibilities? (*Probe:* e.g. for particular groups of children: other responsibilities?)

Yes    1
No    2

**223**

If 'Yes', specify staff and nature of responsibilities.

| Staff | Responsibility |
|-------|----------------|
|       |                |
|       |                |

*Now I would like to discuss a number of decisions and events which crop up in organizing a unit like this. For each of them, think of the last occasion when the decision or event occurred, and tell me about this.*

| | | Source | | Finance | | Choice | |
|---|---|---|---|---|---|---|---|
| 5. | How were new clothes obtained for the children? | Central store | 0 | Requisitioned | 0 | None | 0 |
| | | Specific shop | 1 | Credit | 1 | Limited | 1 |
| | | Any shop | 2 | Cash | 2 | Unlimited | 2 |
| | | Not applicable | X | Not applicable | X | Not applicable | X |
| 6. | How were new toys obtained for the children? | Central store | 0 | Requisitioned | 0 | None | 0 |
| | | Specific shop | 1 | Credit | 1 | Limited | 1 |
| | | Any shop | 2 | Cash | 2 | Unlimited | 2 |
| | | Not applicable | X | Not applicable | X | Not applicable | X |
| 7. | How were supplies of groceries obtained? | Central store | 0 | Requisitioned | 0 | None | 0 |
| | | Specific shop | 1 | Credit | 1 | Limited | 1 |
| | | Any shop | 2 | Cash | 2 | Unlimited | 2 |
| | | Not applicable | X | Not applicable | X | Not applicable | X |
| 8. | How were supplies of greengroceries obtained? | Central store | 0 | Requisitioned | 0 | None | 0 |
| | | Specific shop | 1 | Credit | 1 | Limited | 1 |
| | | Any shop | 2 | Cash | 2 | Unlimited | 2 |
| | | Not applicable | X | Not applicable | X | Not applicable | X |
| 9. | How were supplies of bread obtained? | Central store | 0 | Requisitioned | 0 | None | 0 |
| | | Specific shop | 1 | Credit | 1 | Limited | 1 |
| | | Any shop | 2 | Cash | 2 | Unlimited | 2 |
| | | Not applicable | X | Not applicable | X | Not applicable | X |
| 10. | How was new crockery obtained? | Central store | 0 | Requisitioned | 0 | None | 0 |
| | | Specific shop | 1 | Credit | 1 | Limited | 1 |
| | | Any shop | 2 | Cash | 2 | Unlimited | 2 |
| | | Not applicable | X | Not applicable | X | Not applicable | X |
| 11. | How were cleaning materials obtained? | Central store | 0 | Requisitioned | 0 | None | 0 |
| | | Specific shop | 1 | Credit | 1 | Limited | 1 |
| | | Any shop | 2 | Cash | 2 | Unlimited | 2 |
| | | Not applicable | X | Not applicable | X | Not applicable | X |
| 12. | How were new supplies of linen sheets and towels obtained? | Central store | 0 | Requisitioned | 0 | None | 0 |
| | | Specific shop | 1 | Credit | 1 | Limited | 1 |
| | | Any shop | 2 | Cash | 2 | Unlimited | 2 |
| | | Not applicable | X | Not applicable | X | Not applicable | X |
| 13. | How were soft furnishings obtained? | Central store | 0 | Requisitioned | 0 | None | 0 |
| | | Specific shop | 1 | Credit | 1 | Limited | 1 |
| | | Any shop | 2 | Cash | 2 | Unlimited | 2 |
| | | Not applicable | X | Not applicable | X | Not applicable | X |
| 14. | How were birthday presents obtained? | Central store | 0 | Requisitioned | 0 | None | 0 |
| | | Specific shop | 1 | Credit | 1 | Limited | 1 |
| | | Any shop | 2 | Cash | 2 | Unlimited | 2 |
| | | Not applicable | X | Not applicable | X | Not applicable | X |

15. Do you have a petty cash allowance?     No    0
                                            Yes    1

   If 'Yes', what is it used for?

16. What arrangements are made for the children's holidays?
    (*Probe:* Who chooses place; arranges accommodation, travel, etc.; how is it paid
    for?)

*The following decisions relate to the children. Again, think about the last time the event occurred, but this time, tell me who made the decision.*

| | Final say | | Discuss before with superiors | | Discuss before with subordinates | |
|---|---|---|---|---|---|---|
| 17. Who decided last time that a child should be admitted to the unit? | Superior | 0 | No | 0 | No | 0 |
| | Specialist | 1 | Yes | 2 | Yes | 2 |
| | Head of unit | 2 | | | | |
| | Other | 3 | | | | |
| | D.A. | X | | X | | X |
| 18. Who decided last time a child was ready to attend school/training centre? | Superior | 0 | No | 0 | No | 0 |
| | Specialist | 1 | Yes | 2 | Yes | 2 |
| | Head of unit | 2 | | | | |
| | Other | 3 | | | | |
| | D.A. | X | | X | | X |
| 19. Last time it was necessary to remove a child from the unit? | Superior | 0 | No | 0 | No | 0 |
| | Specialist | 1 | Yes | 2 | Yes | 2 |
| | Head of unit | 2 | | | | |
| | Other | 3 | | | | |
| | D.A. | X | | X | | X |
| 20. Last time a child went on home leave? | Superior | 0 | No | 0 | No | 0 |
| | Specialist | 1 | Yes | 2 | Yes | 2 |
| | Head of unit | 2 | | | | |
| | Other | 3 | | | | |
| | D.A. | X | | X | | X |
| 21. Last time it was necessary for a child to be restrained? | Superior | 0 | No | 0 | No | 0 |
| | Specialist | 1 | Yes | 2 | Yes | 2 |
| | Head of unit | 2 | | | | |
| | Other | 3 | | | | |
| | D.A. | X | | X | | X |
| 22. Last time it was necessary for a child to have special treatment e.g. physiotherapy, etc.? | Superior | 0 | No | 0 | No | 0 |
| | Specialist | 1 | Yes | 2 | Yes | 2 |
| | Head of unit | 2 | | | | |
| | Other | 3 | | | | |
| | D.A. | X | | X | | X |
| 23. Last time a visitor was appointed for a child other than his parents | Superior | 0 | No | 0 | No | 0 |
| | Specialist | 1 | Yes | 2 | Yes | 2 |
| | Head of unit | 2 | | | | |
| | Other | 3 | | | | |
| | D.A. | X | | X | | X |

*And now, just a few questions about decisions affecting the staff:*

| | Final say | | Discuss before with superiors | | Discuss before with subordinates | |
|---|---|---|---|---|---|---|
| 24. Who decided what this week's off-duty should be? | Office | 0 | No | 0 | No | 0 |
| | Unit | 2 | Yes | 2 | Yes | 2 |
| | Other | X | | X | | X |
| 25. Who decided about this/last year's holiday periods | Office | 0 | No | 0 | No | 0 |
| | Unit | 2 | Yes | 2 | Yes | 2 |
| | Other | X | | X | | X |
| 26. Who decided about this week's allocation of tasks to staff? | Office | 0 | No | 0 | No | 0 |
| | Unit | 2 | Yes | 2 | Yes | 2 |
| | Other | X | | X | | X |
| 27. Who decided about the appointment of new members of staff? | Office | 0 | No | 0 | No | 0 |
| | Unit | 2 | Yes | 2 | Yes | 2 |
| | Other | X | | X | | X |

225

Q

*Now, you can tell me if you have been given any regulations from 'the office', or standing orders from your superiors, about the following events:*

|  | Yes | Yes, but discretion | No | Other |
|---|---|---|---|---|
| 28. The time the children get up? | 0 | 1 | 2 | X |
| 29. The time the children go to bed? | 0 | 1 | 2 | X |
| 30. The number of baths the children have? | 0 | 1 | 2 | X |
| 31. The times at which the children are toileted? | 0 | 1 | 2 | X |
| 32. The times at which parents can visit? | 0 | 1 | 2 | X |
| 33. The times at which children have meals? | 0 | 1 | 2 | X |

34. How often is your unit visited by your immediate superior? (probe for regularity and time)

Per day _____
Per week_____
Other _____

35. How often is your unit visited by the doctor (ward or G.P.)? (Pro be for regularity and time)

Per day _____
Per week_____
Other _____

36. Are you ever visited or inspected by anyone else in an official capacity? (e.g. by R.H.B., Local Authority, Board of Governors, etc.)
    Probe:

| Who | Frequency | Last visit | Reason | Evaluation |
|---|---|---|---|---|
|  |  |  |  |  |
|  |  |  |  |  |
|  |  |  |  |  |

37. Are there any regular staff meetings within the establishment?

No 0
Yes 2

If 'Yes', how often are they held? _____
Who goes to them? _____

38. Are there any case conferences or discussions within the establishment?

No 0
Yes 2

If 'Yes', how often are they held? _____
Who goes to them? _____

THANK YOU VERY MUCH FOR YOUR HELP

## Form C4: Staff Questionnaire

One questionnaire was left for each member of staff who had worked in the unit during the week of the fieldwork. An explanatory letter asked for their co-operation, and, where possible, staff were encouraged by the fieldworkers to complete the form. The forms were distributed on the day the research worker left, and a pre-paid, addressed envelope was supplied by the research unit. Eighty-five per cent of staff returned their questionnaires, duly completed.

---

|  |  |
|---|---|
| FORM C4<br>STAFF QUESTIONNAIRE<br><br>STRICTLY CONFIDENTIAL | Office use only<br><br>Estab.<br>Unit<br>Staff |

*This form is for research purposes only, and your answers are confidential. Answer all questions as accurately as you can, either by placing a cross (X) in the appropriate box, or by PRINTING in the space provided. Thank you.*

| | Leave blank | | Leave blank |
|---|---|---|---|
| 1. Grade/status _____ | 2 3<br>4 X | 7. Are you liable to be moved from one ward to another within establishment?<br>No        Yes | 0<br>1<br>X |
| 2. Age: 15–24   25–34<br>       35–44   45–54<br>       55–64   Over<br>              65 | 0 1<br>2 3<br>4 5<br>X | 8. When did you start work in this ward or unit?<br>Date _____ | |
| 3. Sex: Male    Female | 0 1 | 9. When did you start work in this establishment?<br>Date _____ | |
| 4. Marital status:<br>Married<br>Single<br>Widowed<br>Divorced<br>Separated | 0<br>1<br><br>2<br><br>X | 10. How long have you worked with severely subnormal children?<br>Years— Months— Days— | |
| 5. Number of children:<br>Under 16 years _____<br>Over 16 years _____<br>None _____ | | 11. What qualifications do you have? e.g. S.R.N., Home Office Cert., etc.<br><br>_____ | |
| 6. Describe in as much detail as you can your father's occupation:<br>_____ | 0 1<br><br>2 3<br>4 X | | |

12. *Here is a list of activities carried out in wards or units like yours. First, read down the list carefully. Then go through, item by item, and put a cross (X) in column 1 if you usually do that activity as a regular part of your job. Put a cross in column 2 if you sometimes do that activity, e.g. if someone is sick, or you are short of staff, but do not regularly do it. Put a cross in column 3 if you never do it.*

|  | Col. 1 | Col. 2 | Col. 3 | |
|---|---|---|---|---|
|  | Usually | Sometimes | Never | Leave blank |
| 1. Heavy cleaning – polishing, scrubbing, etc. | | | | |
| 2. Light cleaning – dusting, sweeping, etc. | | | | |
| 3. Bed making | | | | |
| 4. Washing children's clothes | | | | |
| 5. Ironing children's clothes | | | | |
| 6. Sluicing soiled linen | | | | |
| 7. Packing, unpacking or checking laundry | | | | |
| 8. Mending or darning children's clothes | | | | |
| 9. Preparing breakfast for children | | | | |
| 10. Preparing midday meal for children | | | | |
| 11. Preparing evening meal for children | | | | |
| 12. Laying or clearing tables | | | | |
| 13. Washing or drying dishes | | | | |
| 14. Getting the children up in the mornings | | | | |

| | Col. 1 | Col. 2 | Col. 3 | |
|---|---|---|---|---|
| | Usually | Sometimes | Never | Leave blank |
| 15. Dressing or undressing children | | | | |
| 16. Washing or bathing children | | | | |
| 17. Toileting or 'changing' children | | | | |
| 18. Feeding children | | | | |
| 19. Serving drinks to children | | | | |
| 20. Playing with the children | | | | |
| 21. Taking children for walks | | | | |
| 22. Nursing sick children | | | | |
| 23. Giving out drugs or medicine | | | | |
| 24. Putting children to bed at night | | | | |
| 25. Attending to children who wake at night | | | | |
| 26. Going to a 'case conference' or discussion | | | | |
| 27. Going to a staff meeting | | | | |
| 28. Discussing children with parents | | | | |
| 29. Discussing children with doctors | | | | |
| 30. Discussing children with teachers | | | | |
| 31. Writing records or reports on the children | | | | |

229

|  | Col. 1 | Col. 2 | Col. 3 |  |
|---|---|---|---|---|
|  | Usually | Sometimes | Never | Leave blank |
| 32. Writing records or reports about the unit |  |  |  |  |
| 33. Filling in requisition forms (for food, clothes, etc.) |  |  |  |  |

Check that for each item you have crossed *one*
of the columns

THANK YOU FOR ALL YOUR HELP

# III  Observation schedules, instructions for use and reliabilities

**Form B2: Observation Check List**

This schedule was completed, at intervals, during several days of observation in each living unit. Some events, such as tea or evening meal activities, were observed and recorded on this form on the afternoons when the Long Day (Staff Activities) Observations were *not* being carried out. Other events were observed in the course of the Long Day Observations and were recorded in summary form on this schedule when time permitted. Much of the data collected in this way was used in the development of scale items. Reliability studies of the observations were carried out by three observers, working in pairs, during the pilot studies, and again by two observers at the end of the fieldwork. Two observers always observed the same events, and each separate observation made by the two observers was compared. Agreed observations were then expressed as a percentage of the total observations. The mean level of agreement was 92·0 per cent. In all, more than forty hours of observations were compared in this way.

| FORM B2<br><br>OBSERVATION CHECK LIST | Office use only<br><br>Estab.<br>Unit |  |
|---|---|---|
| A. MORNING | *Day 1* | *Day 2* |
| 1. What are the ambulant children doing between getting dressed and breakfast? | | |
| Playing | 1 | 1 |
| Getting washed | 2 | 2 |
| Doing nothing | 3 | 3 |
| 2. What are the ambulant children doing immediately before breakfast? | | |
| Lined up or waiting in a group | 1 | 1 |
| Enter dining room in small groups | 2 | 2 |
| Enter dining room individually | 3 | 3 |

231

| | Day 1 | Day 2 |
|---|---|---|
| B. TEA OR EVENING MEAL | | |
| 3. When does first child sit down? | | |
| 4. When does last child sit down? | | |
| 5. When is first child served? | | |
| 6. When is the last child served? | | |
| 7. When does last child finish? | | |
| 8. When does first child begin new activity? | | |
| 9. When does last child begin new activity? | | |
| 10. Describe how table is laid | | |
| 11. Staff eating with children? | | |
|     Yes | 0 | 0 |
|     Yes, sit at tables but do not eat | 1 | 1 |
|     No, supervise standing | 2 | 2 |
| C. TOILETING | | |
| 12. How do ambulant children go to the toilet? (all children) | | |
|     Individually | 0 | 0 |
|     Groups | 1 | 1 |
|     Altogether | 2 | 2 |
| 13. How is toileting organized for those needing help? | | |
|     One staff pots, washes, etc., one child | 0 | 0 |
|     Some children handled by one staff; others by more than one | 1 | 1 |
|     All children handled by more than one staff | 2 | 2 |
| 14. How do ambulant children return from toilet? | | |
|     Individually | 0 | 0 |
|     Groups | 1 | 1 |
|     Altogether | 2 | 2 |
| 15. How many routine toilet sessions are there? | | |
| D. BATHING | | |
| 16. When does this occur? | | |
|     Throughout the day | 0 | 0 |
|     Specific time | 1 | 1 |
| 17. Where are children who are not being bathed? | | |
|     All waiting in bathroom or elsewhere | 0 | 0 |
|     Some waiting in bathroom or elsewhere | 1 | 1 |
|     All playing, etc. elsewhere; go for bath individually | 2 | 2 |
| 18. How do ambulant children return from bathing? | | |
|     Individually | 0 | 0 |
|     Groups | 1 | 1 |
|     Altogether | 2 | 2 |
| 19. How is process organized for those needing help? | | |
|     One staff baths, dries and dresses a child | 0 | 0 |
|     Some children bathed, etc., by more than one person | 1 | 1 |
|     All children bathed, etc., by more than one person | 2 | 2 |

| E. OTHER MATTERS | Day 1 | Day 2 |
|---|---|---|
| 20. Children seen in kitchen? *Number* *Frequency* | | |
| 21. Children seen in other areas? *Note location* | | |
| 22. Do staff sit and watch TV with children? | | |
| Yes, someone sitting all the time | 0 | 0 |
| Yes, someone, some of the time | 1 | 1 |
| Supervise only | 2 | 2 |
| Doesn't apply – no TV | 3 | 3 |
| Other | 4 | 4 |
| 23. Did any go for walks? If so, how were they organized? | | |
| 24. Did any go into yard or garden? | | |
| 25. Between what times were children observed playing (check Form C2)? | | |
| 26. Where are private clothes kept? | | |
| 27. Where are private toys kept? | | |
| 28. Where are daily clothes kept? | | |
| 29. Are daily clothes marked with names? | | |
| 30. No. of rooms with pictures, pin-ups, etc.? | | |

The last five items may be observed after children go to bed.

## Form C2: Long Day [Staff Activities] Observations

This recording schedule was used by the fieldworker to record the activities of staff and certain aspects of their interaction with children during systematic observations conducted on a time sampling basis. The observations related to the head of the unit, junior child care staff and domestic staff, during two mornings and two afternoons and evenings in the week of the fieldwork. Observations in each living unit totalled more than nineteen hours over two days.

## Reliability between observers

Observer reliabilities, according to Bijou *et al.* (1969), are dependent upon (1) the adequacy of the observational codes, (2) the training of observers, (3) the frequency of observations over sessions (time sampling) and (4) the method of calculating reliability coefficients. We can deal with the first two points together.

In general, the more specific, exhaustive and mutually exclusive the codes are, the more reliable will be the results – but only if the observers are adequately trained. The schedule was developed after extensive pilot work in two children's wards of a large subnormality hospital, two residential nurseries for normal children and one Local Authority hostel for the retarded, none of which were included in the later survey. Three fieldworkers were involved in the pilot institutions, working singly and in pairs. In the early stages of the pilot, which lasted for several weeks and involved many scores of hours of observation, the fieldworkers worked in relays so that the period from the time the children got up, until the time they went to bed, was fully covered (hence the title Long Day Observations). During this period, many different events were observed – lists of activities for coding were devised and the reliability with which they could be observed was checked. Fieldworkers repeatedly discussed the results and modified the coding systems until satisfactory levels of reliability were reached. This period provided an intensive training period for the observers, and also produced a detailed list of activities and events for coding purposes. The final instructions for fieldworkers and the denotative definitions for coding are reproduced at the end of this appendix.

For each member of staff, it was finally decided to record the following information during each observation interval: her activity; whether or not children were present during the activity; if children were present, whether or not interaction between them and the staff member took place, and particularly if the member of staff spoke to them; and finally a rating of the quality of any interaction according to whether the member of staff concerned was rejecting, tolerating or accepting towards the children. (We also recorded where the activity took place and whether staff talked to each other during the interval, but in the event neither of these observations seemed worthy of extensive analysis.)

There were a number of considerations involved in selecting the time samples for observing these activities. First, it was not possible to select arbitrary time periods because it was probable that the pattern of staff activities followed a natural history throughout the day, according to the nature of the routine. To compare two units from 3 p.m. to 4 p.m. would clearly have been misleading if, in one unit, it was bath-time, and in another it was tea-time. It was therefore decided to observe 'functional periods', that is, to observe a whole sequence of activity, regardless of how long it took, subject to certain maximum limits. We observed, for example, from the time the children got up until the time they went to school, because it was clear from the pilot enquiries that certain activities would be bound to occur in all units during that time. Second, we wished to be as sure as we could that we were not observing an atypical occasion. Observations were therefore spread out over four of the five days' fieldwork with two mornings and two afternoons and evenings being observed. It was thus possible to compare the same unit on different occasions, to assess the typicality of the observations. In the event, the findings from the second set of observations almost exactly repeated those from the first set of observations in all units. Third, we wished to find an observation and recording interval, in which only one observation of each event would be possible. It was found, during the pilot, that even a ten-second interval was too long for this purpose in the residential nurseries, and that an interval of a minute or longer might have been short enough for the hospitals at certain times of the day. A thirty-second interval was found to be the most appropriate compromise.

The method for calculating the reliability coefficient was the most stringent of those discussed by Bijou et al. (1969). The same technique was used for assessing reliability of the other instruments used in these studies.

The procedure was as follows. Observers worked two at a time and observed the same situation from the same location. To avoid the problem of stop-watches becoming out of synchronization, observers stood next to each other and used the same watch. Subsequently, reliability studies were conducted with separate watches, with only a marginal loss in reliability, possibly because the observation interval was relatively long. The recording schedules of the two observers were then compared: events had to occur in the same interval on both recording schedules to be counted as agreement; any events recorded as occuring in different intervals on the two schedules, and any omissions, were counted as errors. Agreed observations were then expressed as a proportion of the total observations (agreed + disagreed) to give the reliability coefficient. Reliability coefficients were calculated for each column, representing a class of events, on the schedule. Bijou discusses the possibility that even with this technique, reliability can appear meaninglessly high if the event to be observed is of extremely low frequency. In that case, observers are simply agreed that something did *not* happen. Since none of the events we observed had such low frequencies, and in each interval *something* had to be coded, our reliability coefficients are not inflated in that way.

Not surprisingly, reliability improved during the course of the pilot,

TABLE III.1 *Reliability coefficients: long day (staff activities) observations*

| | Staff activity codes | Presence of children | Interaction occurrence | Talk | Interaction evaluation |
|---|---|---|---|---|---|
| **Pilot studies** | | | | | |
| *Nurseries* | | | | | |
| Observers 2 and 3 | 66·2 | 100·0 | 74·8 | 98·5 | 92·7 |
| Observers 1 and 3 | 74·0 | 100·0 | 80·5 | 98·6 | 75·3 |
| Observers 2 and 3 | 80·4 | 96·4 | 86·1 | 90·4 | 84·5 |
| *Hospital wards* | | | | | |
| Observers 1 and 2 | 93·3 | 97·3 | 88·0 | 85·3 | 62·7 |
| Observers 1 and 2 | 84·8 | 100·0 | 84·8 | 93·5 | 67·4 |
| Observers 1 and 3 | 94·4 | 91·7 | 77·8 | 88·9 | 58·3 |
| *Hostel* | | | | | |
| Observers 2 and 3 | 88·6 | 94·9 | 85·9 | 92·4 | 68·4 |
| *Conclusion of survey* | | | | | |
| *Hospital wards* | | | | | |
| Observers 1 and 2 | 98·0 | 97·5 | 99·2 | 95·8 | 90·0 |
| Observers 1 and 2 | 97·4 | 100·0 | 98·2 | 97·4 | 93·2 |

as definitions became accepted and the fieldworkers more experienced. Once the final form was established, a further reliability check was run in each of the pilot institutions. Because it was feared, for various reasons, that reliability might decline as the main study progressed, a final reliability check was made between Observers 1 and 2, who actually conducted the survey, at the end of the fieldwork. The reliability coefficients are given in Table III.1.

It can be seen from Table III.1 that the level of agreement for all these classes of events was generally high, although it was higher between Observers 1 and 2 than between Observers 1 and 3 or 2 and 3. The reliability coefficients for the presence of children and the incidence of talk never fell below 85 per cent. The coefficient for staff activities twice fell below 80 per cent, both times involving Observer 3 and both times in a residential nursery, where it was acknowledged that the observation interval was too long. The coefficient for the occurrence of staff-child interaction fell below 80 per cent only once, again in a residential nursery. It was inevitable that the coefficient for the evaluation of interaction would be lower than the others, since this was the only observation which involved the qualitative judgment of the observer. Even so, the level of agreement was acceptably high, and at the end of the fieldwork there appeared to have been some improvement in the reliability with which observers evaluated interaction. (We did try to evaluate various other events, such as the warmth and direction of talk, during the pilot, but we were unable to do this with an acceptable level of reliability.)

The recording schedule, and instructions for its completion, are given below.

# OBSERVATION SCHEDULES, INSTRUCTIONS FOR USE AND RELIABILITIES

FORM C2

LONG DAY OBSERVATIONS

(STAFF ACTIVITIES)

For office use

Estab. ☐ Unit ☐
Date ☐ ☐ ☐
Sheet No. _____

Time began

| 1 S | 2 Acti- vity | 3 Code | 4 S-C inter- action | 5 C | 6 R | 7 Tol. | 8 A | 9 T | 10 Loc. | 11 No. of C. | 12 No. of S. | 13 ST | Analy- sis |
|---|---|---|---|---|---|---|---|---|---|---|---|---|---|
| | | | | | | | | | | | | | |
| Head of unit | | | | | | | | | | | | | |
| | | | | | | | | | | | | | |
| | | | | | | | | | | | | | |
| Child care staff | | | | | | | | | | | | | |
| | | | | | | | | | | | | | |
| | | | | | | | | | | | | | |
| Domes- tic staff | | | | | | | | | | | | | |
| | | | | | | | | | | | | | |

237

## Rules for the Conduct of Long Day Observations

1. From staff time-table (Form C1), ascertain who will be on duty on day of observations. (Be sure to check this before observations begin.)
2. Divide staff into three role groups: head of unit, child care staff, domestic staff. Each C2 sheet covers a 15-minute cycle of observations, 5 minutes for each role group. The head of unit is always observed first in each cycle. There will be usually only one head of unit – though some hospital wards operating a shift system may have two heads of units on at the same time for a short period. If so, observe them in alternating 15-minute cycles. Child care staff will probably include several members. Before observations begin, list them and select a random sequence for observing. Observe only one member of the role group in each 15-minute cycle. There may be several domestic staff also. If so, decide a random sequence and observe as for child care staff.
3. Each 15-minute cycle is spent as follows. Head of the unit is observed for three 30-second intervals, each of which is followed by a 30-second interval for recording; three minutes have now elapsed and two minutes are now spent locating the relevant member of child care staff. Child care staff observed for three 30-second intervals, followed by three 30-second recording periods. Two minutes to locate relevant domestic staff. Three 30-second observations of domestic staff, followed by three 30-second recording periods. Two minutes to locate head of unit. Cycle begins again.
4. Time of commencing each sheet *must* be marked in space provided.
5. Number of each sheet *must* be marked in space provided.
6. First space on each sheet *ONLY* for head of unit.
   Second space on each sheet *ONLY* for child care staff.
   Third space on each sheet *ONLY* for domestic staff.
7. Intervals between observations within role groups must be exactly 30 seconds; in difficult circumstances, stick to this as closely as possible (e.g. if somebody has moved while recording, it might take longer).
8. Actual observation periods must be exactly 30 seconds.
9. Intervals between observing one role group and another may be flexible, but usually two minutes. If longer intervals occur for any reason, make a note of this on the schedule.
10. If any role group is unrepresented (i.e. no one is on duty from that group) at the time of observation, go on immediately to the next role group, in a 10-minute cycle instead of a 15-minute cycle. (Usually, it will be domestics at the beginning and end of the day who are not on duty.) Exceptionally only one role group may be on duty, and here, a 5-minute cycle should be used. Mark space for role groups who are off duty as OFF DUTY.
11. If, on the other hand, a particular representative of a role group is on duty, but cannot be located, do not reduce the cycle, but use all of the available time (two minutes' location and three minutes' observation time) to find them. If they are found within this time, observe them as normally, even if this means the cycle is extended to twenty minutes. If they are not found within this time, select a substitute from the same role group and observe, or if no substitute available, mark that role group as ABSENT.

## Completing the Recording Schedule

*Col. 1.* 'S' Give clear indication of who is being observed.

*Col. 2 'Activity'* A brief description of the activity *must be given in all cases*, so that a check can be made on codes in Col. 3. This is especially important where there is any doubt about coding.

*Col. 3.* '*Code*' Only the following codes are to be used:

    A = administrative

    D = domestic

    CF = 'functional' (i.e. physical) child care

    CS = social child care

    S = supervisory

    M = miscellaneous

These codes must be used strictly in accordance with the attached sheet of denotative definitions. In some cases, more than one code might be necessary per half-minute interval; record as in the following example:

    Makes beds  D

    Takes a child to toilet  CF

As a general rule, do not break down activities in smaller sub-activities unless the first activity has definitely stopped and a new one begun. For instance, if – while making beds – a nurse is also talking to the children as she does so, record D in column 3 and note the interaction in columns 4 and 5.

If an activity cannot be coded on the spot for any reason, put a '?' in column 3, and make sure there is an adequate description of the activity in column 2.

*Col. 4.* '*S-C Interaction*' A brief description of the interaction between staff and children should be given here. If possible, record comments made and the quality of the interaction. Use this column for *any* interaction which occurs within the interval *regardless* of the main activity. If there is no interaction, write 'none'.

*Col. 5.* '*C*' This column is to be used only where A, D, M or S have been coded in column 3. Put a tick in column 5 wherever activities coded as A, D, M or S have involved interaction with the children. Put a cross in column 5 wherever activities coded A, D, M or S did not involve interaction with the children. If the only activity has been coded as CF or CS, then there should be no entry in column 5. If there is more than one entry in column 3, e.g. D/CF/A, then there could be two ticks or crosses or one tick and one cross in column 5, according to whether D or A involved interaction. This column should then tell us whether in situations other than CF or CS, each activity involved interaction.

*Cols. 6, 7* and *8.* '*R*', '*Tol.*', '*A*' The definitions of each category are given below. Only *one* tick should appear in *one* of the three columns for each time period. During the observation period, several types of interaction may have occurred; in this case, take the highest, most favourable rating which occurred during the time period and tick that column. These colums will thus show the most favourable interaction which occurred in each time period, in the same way as talking (column 9) does. No borderlines are permitted; if doubtful, put a '?' in the most appropriate column.

If no interaction is possible throughout the 30-second interval, because no children are present, draw a horizontal line through the three columns. If any children are present for any part of the time, or all of the time, one tick only must be recorded in one of the three columns.

*R = rejects (or ignores)*: if no interaction is initiated by staff (verbal or non-verbal) this counts as ignores. If children initiate interaction by speaking, making noises, tugging at sleeve, or in any other way, and the staff make no response at all, or push the child away, or respond negatively by saying 'don't do that', or otherwise telling the child off without further interaction, count this as rejecting.

*Tol. = tolerates*: if staff initiates interaction which is functional – 'do this'; 'get down'; 'go to the toilet', then this counts as toleration. If child initiates interaction in any way and is not fended off or told off, but receives some simple

239

acknowledgment which is sufficient for the situation, but not positive, count this as 'tolerates'.

*A = accepts:* If staff initiate social interaction, playful remarks, poking, tickling, patting, etc., or – when child approaches them – they stop what they are doing to respond in a positive or playful way, then count this as 'accepts'.

Note that play situations can be rated as 'Rejecting' and non-play situations can be rated as 'Accepting'.

*Col. 9. 'T'* Put a tick if there is any talking to the children at all during the observation interval. Only one tick per time interval is allowed. If there was no talking, put a cross. If you were not sure, put a '?'.

*Columns 4-9 inclusive should be filled in only if children are present for at least part of the interval. If no children are present for the whole interval. draw a horizontal line extending through columns 4, 5, 6, 7, 8 and 9.*

*Col. 10. 'Loc.'* Put a clear indication of the location of the staff member for each of the activities which are coded in column 3. This may mean several locations. Do not include locations which are only passed through, unless some specific activity has been recorded in that location.

*Col. 11. 'No. of C.'* Put a clear indication of the approximate number or proportion (in small units it should be possible to get exact numbers) of the children present in each location for which an activity has been recorded. If children are in the doorway, or just outside the room, but are *clearly* within an *actual* interaction situation (e.g. being spoken to through a serving hatch), count them as present.

*Col. 12. 'No. of S.'* If the head of unit is being observed, this column refers to presence or absence of junior staff, whose numbers for each activity recorded should be noted. If other staff are being observed, the presence or absence of the head of unit for each activity should be recorded.

*Col. 13. 'ST'* If the head of unit speaks to, or is spoken to by, junior staff, this should be marked with a tick. Talking between junior staff and talking to outsiders does not count. Only one tick allowed per observation interval.

*Before returning forms to the office for filing,* the following procedure must be observed:

1. Check that each sheet is numbered and timed.
2. Check that each role group is clearly marked.
3. Identify each individual observation period by numbering observations.
4. Check that every column has been correctly filled in according to the above procedures.
5. Ring in pencil any queries or doubts which cannot be resolved and make a list of those on a separate piece of paper.
6. Tie the whole batch of observations together in the following order: 1st morning, 1st afternoon, 2nd morning, 2nd afternoon, with the separate sheet attached. Mark clearly on the separate sheet the time periods actually observed, the date of the observations, the unit and institution numbers and the name of the observer.

## Use of activity codes

1. If two or more activities occur simultaneously (usually this will mean supervising other children while engaged in something else – e.g. at tea-time or watching others while bathing child), record only the main activity; in these examples, ignore the supervising aspect.
2. If two or more distinct activities occur in sequence during an interval, use two or more codes. However, if one activity is clearly preparatory to something

else which takes place within the interval, code only the latter. E.g. gets toys from cupboard and then plays with children – code only CS. If whole interval was spent in getting toys from cupboard, code D. If a main activity is broken off and a minor one occurs within it, use two or more codes; e.g. if playing with children on floor, stops to prevent a child running out of the door, then returns to playing, code CS.S.CS. Again, if sitting at table serving a meal, and has to retrieve child who had got down from table, code CF.S.

3. The supervision category is to be used in effect only if no other major activity is going on at the same time. The only exceptions to this are when the supervision itself is a discreet activity, e.g. restraining a child, sending a child somewhere, and where staff are also talking to each other and supervising, then record S rather than M.

4. Remember that every time an activity code is recorded, you must have a corresponding entry under location and number of children. Wherever M.A.D.S. are coded under activity, you must have a tick or cross under the interaction code, if children were present.

*Denotative definitions of Activity Codes*

*1. Domestic Activities: Code D*

Cleaning, polishing floors, etc.
Washing objects
Tidying objects
Folding up and putting away clothes or other materials
Making beds
Lining up beds
Taking things out of cupboards – only if this takes up the whole interval. If, within the interval, staff go on to use the thing, then code whole sequence according to its use
Putting things away in cupboards – again, only if it takes up whole period. If previously within interval it has been used, code whole as according to use
Opening or closing windows, curtains, etc.
Dusting, etc.
Hanging up coats, etc.
Ironing
Sluicing soiled materials
Packing, unpacking laundry or similar activities
Mending or darning
Preparing food (away from the table – i.e. do not include dishing up, serving, or handing out, or collecting food)
Washing up
Drying up
Cooking food
Laying table before meal ⎫ exclude taking away or giving out things
Clearing table after meal ⎭ within the meal
Clearing up after play – exclude adjustments to sand trays, water, etc., during play
Looking for bath plugs, taps, etc.
Untying cots and nets
Locking doors, etc.

*2. Functional Child Care: Code CF*

Getting children up
Putting children on/off toilets, pots, etc.

241

R

Wiping bottoms, noses, etc.
Bathing/drying children
Running or letting out of bath water as part of the bathing process
Hair combing or washing
Putting children to bed
Tucking them in
Pulling back bedclothes when children are getting into or out of bed
Dressing or undressing children
Feeding, actually assisting in process
Teeth-cleaning
Washing/drying children
Cutting up food for children
Pouring out drinks
Serving out food of any kind, including sweets
Dishing food up on to plates
Handing out plates or collecting them back during a meal
Tying laces
Getting flannels, towels, clothes, etc., for children preparatory to use
Giving out medicines
Giving nursing attention of any kind
Taking children to and from toilets, bathroom, etc., if actually involved in the
    toileting or washing
Asking a child if he wants more of something
Moving spastic children
Saying good morning to the children
Putting on bibs and aprons
Pushing chair with child on it
Saying goodbye to children
Taking children to school
Examining sick child
Pushing children's chairs under table, children sitting on them
Saying Grace at tables

### 3. *Social Child Care: Code CS*

Playing any kind of formal or informal game with children or amusing them
Reading stories
Teasing
Singing with or to children
Playing musical instruments
Educational activities and games
Reading a letter to a child
Taking children for a walk
Handling play material with or for the benefit of children during or preparatory
    to play situation
Giving a child a piggy-back
Going off on a trip
Looking out of windows and taking an interest in things with children
Watching television with children and sitting down with them
Showing children how to do something

### 4. *Administration: Code A*

Paper work of any kind – registers, medical records, record books, charts,
    laundry lists, time-tables, etc.
Answering 'phone

242

Dealing with visitors to ward of any kind – doctors, professional visitors, parents, other staff, laundrymen, milkmen, etc.

Talking to people – junior staff or others – about administrative or unit matters

Giving instructions to junior staff or directing staff activities within the unit

Junior staff asking senior staff for instructions or receiving them

Putting children's money away

Getting the post

Checking stocks of various kinds

## 5. Supervisory: Code S

Supervising movement of children from one room to another

Supervising toileting, bathing, washing children, etc., where not actually involved physically in the toileting, etc. itself

Watching staff or children carrying out activities

Giving instructions to the children – 'don't do this, or that'; telling them off, however mildly: telling them to get things; calling them back from somewhere, etc.

Directing the management of one group of children by another group of children

Switching television on and off

Standing watching television

Standing watching television with the children

Attending assemblies

Restraining children from going off somewhere, fighting, doing various activities

Interfering in another situation to prevent children from harming selves or others

Sitting at table apart from table at which children sit

Walking around in yard with children to be coded unless they are definitely playing

Handing plates to children to lay table or to give to others

Standing waiting with a child

Taking a child from one place to another

Tying child into chair, etc.

## 6. Miscellaneous: Code M

Chit-chat between staff (when they are not doing anything else, e.g. administration or supervision). If other staff talking cannot be heard, code as M

Staff eating

Staff talk to observers

Staff in toilet, washing hands, etc., and not supervising children

Playing with animals

Staff moving from one place to another

### Long Day Observations, Procedural Instructions

These instructions must be adhered to as closely as possible to ensure an adequate number of observations and to ensure comparability between institutions. Do not stop for tea breaks other than those specified *unless all* staff stop for a break and you are invited to join them. If tea is forced on you at other times, make the break as short as possible.

1. Before Long Day starts, find out: (a) who gets the children up and at what time; (b) what time day staff come on duty; (c) what time children go to and

return from school, and whether any children remain behind in the units; (d) what time all of the children go to bed.

2. Arrive in unit fifteen minutes before children start getting up, and ask night nurse about potting, etc., for management scale. Observe getting up process for management scale until the day staff arrive. If children are got up by day staff, and there are no night staff, management scale observations must be noted while Long Day observations of day staff are being carried out.

3. Start Long Day observations as soon as first member of day staff arrives on duty. Observe role groups in strict rotation continuously for two hours, unless *all* the children have left the unit for school within this time period. If the night nurse overlaps in duty with day staff, include him or her in child care role group. If all of the children have left the unit before the two hours are up, stop observing – see definitions in note 5.

4. After two-hour period, take a fifteen-minute break.

5. After fifteen-minute break, observe continuously until 10.30 a.m. or until *all* the children have left for school if this occurs before the period has elapsed. (If *all* have left before 10.30, stop observing when they leave. If *all* usually go, but for some reason, such as dysentery, they remain on unit, stop observing at time they should have left. If the only children remaining on the unit are sick or bedfast, stop observing at the time the others leave for school. So long as there are *any* ambulant children on the unit, who do not normally go to school, keep observing until 10.30 a.m.)

6. At 10.30, take a break until a few minutes before 11 a.m.

7. At 11 a.m. return to unit, and observe for one hour until 12 noon if there are any ambulant children on the unit.

8. At 12 noon, take a two-hour break until a few minutes before 2 p.m.

9. At 2 p.m. return to unit and observe for one hour until 3 p.m. if there are any ambulant children on the unit.

10. At 3 p.m., take a break until a few minutes before the children return from school. If no children have been to school, or if only a few have been to school and do not return until after 4 p.m., return to unit at 3.55 p.m., ready to start observing at 4 p.m.

11. Start observing again as soon as children return from school (or, where this does not apply, at 4 p.m.) and observe continuously for two hours, unless all children are in bed before time period has elapsed. If they are all in bed within two hours, stop observing when last child is in bed.

12. After a two-hour period (where no schoolchildren, this will be at 6 p.m.) take a fifteen-minute break.

13. After fifteen-minute break, observe continuously until 8 p.m., or until *all* the children are in bed, whichever is the sooner.

# References

*Figures in square brackets indicate pages where these references are cited.*

ADAMS, R. N. (1968), 'Cultural aspects of infantile malnutrition and mental development', 465–74 in SCRIMSHAW, N. S. and GORDON, J. E. (eds), (1968). [39]

AINSWORTH, M. D. *et al.* (1962), *Deprivation of Maternal Care: A reassessment of its effects*, Geneva: WHO [30, 31]

ANASTASI, A. and FOLEY, J. P. (1949), *Differential Psychology*, New York: MacMillan. [26]

ARNASON, B. B. (1958), 'Care and cure as functions of the public mental hospital', unpublished Ph.D. thesis, Cambridge, Mass.: Radcliffe College. [38]

BAKWIN, H. (1942), 'Loneliness in infants', *Amer. J. Dis. Child.*, 63, 30. [31]

BAKWIN, H. (1949), 'Emotional deprivation in infants', *J. Pediat.*, 35, 512. [31]

BARRABEE, P. S. (1951), 'A study of a mental hospital: The effect of its social structure on its functions', unpublished Ph.D. thesis, Harvard University. [38]

BELKNAP, I. (1956), *Human Problems of a State Mental Hospital*, New York: McGraw-Hill. [38, 39, 40]

BERNSTEIN, B. (1970), 'Education cannot compensate for society', *New Society*, 26 Feb. 1970, 344–7. [29]

BETTELHEIM, B. (1959), *Love is not Enough*, London, Collier-MacMillan. [33]

BIJOU, S. W. *et al.* (1969), 'Methodology for experimental studies of young children in natural settings' (mimeographed). [233, 234]

BIRCH, H. G. and GUSSOW, J. D. (1970), *Disadvantaged Children: Health and nutrition*, New York: Grune & Stratton. [28]

BLATT, B. (1967), *Christmas in Purgatory: A photographic essay on mental retardation*, Boston: Allyn & Bacon. [28]

BLATT, B. (1969), 'Purgatory', 37–49, in KUGEL, R. B. and WOLFENSBERGER, W. (eds) (1969). [28]

BLAU, P. M. and SCOTT, W. R. (1963), *Formal Organisations: A comparative approach*, London: Routledge & Kegan Paul. [36]

BOWLBY, J. (1951), *Maternal Care and Mental Health*, Geneva: WHO. [30, 31, 32, 33]

BROWN, R. K. (1967), 'Research and consultancy in industrial enterprises', *Sociology*, 1, 1, 33–60. [38]

BUHLER, C. (1935), *From Birth to Maturity*, London: Kegan Paul. [32]

**245**

# REFERENCES

BURLINGHAM, D. and FREUD, A. (1942), *Young Children in Wartime*, London: Allen & Unwin. [31, 32]

BURLINGHAM, D. and FREUD, A. (1943), *Infants Without Families*, London: Allen & Unwin. [31, 32]

CAUDILL, W. (1958), *The Psychiatric Hospital as a Small Society*, Cambridge, Mass.: Harvard Univ. Press. [38]

*Children in the Care of Local Authorities in England and Wales*, 1953, 1954, 1959, 1963, 1966, Command papers, London: HMSO. [12]

CLARKE, A. D. B. (1965), 'Genetic and environmental studies of intelligence', 92–137 in CLARKE, A. M. and CLARKE, A. D. B. (eds) (1965). [26]

CLARKE, A. D. B. (1968), 'Learning and mental development', *Brit. J. Psychiat.*, 114, 1061–78. [28]

CLARKE, A. M. and CLARKE, A. D. B. (eds) (1965), *Mental Deficiency: The changing outlook*, London: Methuen. [26]

CLEMMER, D. (1940), *The Prison Community*, Boston: Holt, Rinehart & Winston. [36]

COSER, R. L. (1962), *Life on the Ward*, Michigan: State Univ. Press. [135]

CUMMING, J. and CUMMING, E. (1956), 'The locus of power in a large mental hospital', *Psychiatry*, 19, 4, 361–69. [39, 40, 41]

CUMMING, J. and CUMMING, E. (1962), *Ego and Milieu*, New York: Atherton. [38, 39, 41]

CURTIS, M. (Chairman) (1946), *Report of the Care of Children Committee*, London: HMSO., Command 6922. [8, 9, 10, 12, 13, 14, 16, 21, 23, 116, 201]

DAVIES, S. P. (1939), *Social Control of the Mentally Deficient*, New York: Cromwell. [23]

DENTLER, R. A. and MACKLER, B. (1961), 'The socialisation of retarded children in an institution', *J. of Health and Human Behav.*, 2, 243–52. [37]

DINITZ, S., LEFTON, M. and PASAMANICK, B. (1959), 'Status perception in a mental hospital', *Social Forces*, 38, 2, 124–8. [39]

DINNAGE, R. and PRINGLE, M. K. (1967), *Residential Child Care: Facts and fallacies*, London: Longmans. [33]

DONNISON, D. V. and UNGERSON, C. (1968), 'Trends in residential care, 1911–1961', *Soc. and Econ. Admin.*, 1968, 2, 75–91. [12]

DUNHAM, H. W. and WEINBERG, S. K. (1960), *The Culture of the State Mental Hospital*, Detroit: Wayne State Univ. Press. [38, 40]

DURFEE, H. and WOLF, K. (1933), in *Z. Kinderforsch*, 42, 273, cited in BOWLBY (1951). [31]

EGGLESTON, S. J. (1967), *The Social Context of the School*, London: Routledge & Kegan Paul. [37]

EISENBERG, L. and CONNERS, C. K. (1968), 'The effect of Head Start on developmental processes', 116–22 in JERVIS, G. A. (ed.) (1968). [28]

ELLIS, N. R. (ed.) (1968), *International Review of Research in Mental Retardation*, 3, New York: Academic Press. [26, 27]

Ely Hospital Inquiry (1969), *Report of the Committee of Inquiry into Allegations of Ill-Treatment of Patients and Other Irregularities at the Ely Hospital, Cardiff*, National Health Service, Command 3975, London: HMSO. [149, 200, 201, 202]

ESHER, F. J. S. (1962), 'On hostels for the subnormal', in *Proc. Int. Copenhagen Cong. for Sci. Stud. of Ment. Retard.*, 2, 690–92. [37]

ETZIONI, A. (1960), 'Interpersonal and structural factors in the study of mental hospitals', *Psychiatry*, 23, 1, 17. [38]

ETZIONI, A. (1961), *A Comparative Analysis of Complex Organisations*, London: Collier-Macmillan. [36, 41]

EYSENCK, H. J. (1960), *The Structure of Human Personality* (2nd edition), London: Methuen. [47]

FALCONER, D. S. (1966), 'Genetic consequences of selection pressure', 219–32 in MEADE, J. E. and PARKES, A. S. (eds) (1966). [26]

FLINT, B. M. (1967), *The Child and the Institution*, London: Univ. of London Press. [37]

FREIDSON, E. (1963), 'Medical sociology; a trend report', *Current Sociol.*, 10–11. [37]

GESELL, A. and ARMATRUDA, C. (1947), *Developmental Diagnosis: Normal and abnormal development. Clinical methods and paediatric applications*, New York: Hoeker. [31]

GOFFMAN, E. (1961), *Asylums: Essays on the social situation of mental patients and other inmates*, New York: Doubleday. [36, 37, 45, 46, 47, 104, 105, 115]

GOOCH, S. and PRINGLE, M. L. K. (1967), 'The interaction of four status variables and measured intelligence and their effect on attainment in two junior schools', *Educational Sciences*, 2, 1, 37–46. [37]

GORDON, H. (1923), *Mental and Scholastic Tests among Retarded Children*, London: HMSO, Board of Education Pamphlet No. 44. [28]

GREENBLATT, M., LEVINSON, D. J. and WILLIAMS, R. H. (eds) (1957), *The Patient and the Mental Hospital*, London: Collier-Macmillan. [38]

GREENBLATT, M., YORK, R. H. and BROWN, E. L. (1955), *From Custodial to Therapeutic Care in Mental Hospitals*, New York: Russell Sage Foundation. [38, 39, 40]

GROSS, N. (1956), 'Sociology of education, 1954–55', in ZETTERBERG, H. L. (ed.) (1956). [37]

GRUENBERG, E. M. (ed.) (1966), 'Evaluating the effectiveness of the mental health services', *Millbank Memorial Fund Quarterly*, 44, 1. [37]

GUSKIN, S. L. and SPICKER, H. H. (1968), 'Educational research in mental retardation', 217–78 in ELLIS, N. R. (ed.), (1968). [26, 27]

HALL, R. H. (1963a), 'Bureaucracy and small organisations', *Sociology and Social Research*, 48, 1, 38–46. [47]

HALL, R. H. (1963b), 'The concept of bureaucracy: an empirical assessment', *Amer. J. Sociol.*, 69, 1, 32–40. [47]

HALL, R. H., HAAS, J. E. and JOHNSON, N. J. (1967), 'An examination of the Blau–Scott and Etzioni typologies', *Admin. Sci. Q.*, 12, 1, 118–39. [36]

HARGREAVES, D. H. (1967), *Social Relations in a Secondary School*, London: Routledge & Kegan Paul. [37]

HENRY, J. (1954), 'The formal social structure of a psychiatric hospital', *Psychiatry*, 17, 2, 139–51. [39]

HENRY, J. (1957), 'Types of institutional structure', in GREENBLATT, M., LEVINSON, D. J. and WILLIAMS, R. H. (eds), (1957). [39]

HEYWOOD, J. S. (1959), *Children in Care*, London: Routledge & Kegan Paul. [5]

HOLLY, D. N. (1965), 'Profiting from a comprehensive school: Class, sex and ability', *Brit. J. Sociol.*, 16, 2, 150–57. [37]

*Hospital Plan for England and Wales* (1962), Command 1604, London: HMSO. [16]

HUNT, J. MCV. (1961), *Intelligence and Experience*, New York: Ronald Press. [26]

HUNTLEY, R. M. C. (1966), 'Heritability of intelligence', 201–18 in MEADE, J. E. and PARKES, A. S. (eds). [26]

HUSEN, T. (1951), 'The influence of schooling upon I.Q.', *Theoria*, 17, 61–88. [28]

HYDE, R. W. and SOLOMON, H. C. (1950), 'Patient government: a new form of group therapy', *Digest of Neurology and Psychiatry*, 18, 207–18. [38]

JENKINS, R. L. (1961), 'A preliminary report on the Psychiatric Evaluation Project', *Co-op. Stud. Psychiat. Res.*, 6, 361–6. [41]

JENKINS, R. L. and GUREL, L. (1959), 'Predictive factors in early release', *Ment. Hosp.*, 10, 11–14. [41]

JENSEN, A. R. (1969), 'How much can we boost I.Q. and scholastic achievement?', *Harvard Educational Review*, 39, 1–123. [26]

JERVIS, G. A. (ed.), (1968), *Expanding Concepts in Mental Retardation*, Springfield, Ill.: C. C. Thomas. [28]

JONES, K. and SIDEBOTHAM, R. (1962), *Mental Hospitals at Work*, London: Routledge & Kegan Paul. [41]

JONES, M. (1953), *The Therapeutic Community*, London: Tavistock Publications. [38]

JONES, M. (1968), *Beyond the Therapeutic Community*, New Haven and London: Yale Univ. Press. [38]

KANNER, L. (1964), *A History of the Care and Study of the Mentally Retarded*, Springfield, Ill.: C. C. Thomas. [23]

KING, R. D. (1970), 'A comparative study of residential care for handicapped children', unpublished Ph.D. thesis, Univ. of London. [72]

KING, R. D. and RAYNES, N. V. (1968a), 'An operational measure of inmate management in residential institutions', *Soc. Sci. and Med.*, 2, 1, 41–53. [64, 109, 112, 207]

KING, R. D. and RAYNES, N. V. (1968b), 'Patterns of institutional care for the severely subnormal', *Amer. J. Ment. Defic.*, 72, 5, 700–9. [95]

KING, R. D. and RAYNES, N. V. (1968c), 'Some determinants of patterns of residential care', 642–9, in *Proc. 1st Cong. Int. Assoc. Sci. Stud. Ment. Defic.*, *Montpellier*, Surrey: Michael Jackson [108, 150].

KIRK, S. A. (1958), *Early Education of the Mentally Retarded*, Urbana, Ill.: Univ. of Illinois Press. [26, 27]

KUGEL, R. B. and WOLFENSBERGER, W. (eds), (1969), *Changing Patterns in Residential Services for the Mentally Retarded*, Washington D.C.: President's Panel on Mental Retardation. [28]

KUSHLICK, A. (1965), 'Community services for the mentally subnormal: A plan for experimental evaluation, *Proc. Roy. Soc. Med.*, 58, 5, 374–80. [142]

KUSHLICK, A. (1968), 'The Wessex Plan for evaluating the effectiveness of residential care for the severely subnormal, 650 in *Proc. 1st Int. Cong. Sci. Stud. Ment. Defic.*, *Montpellier*, Surrey: Michael Jackson. [203]

KUSHLICK, A. and COX, G. (1968), 'The ascertained prevalence of mental subnormality in the Wessex region on 1st July, 1963', 661 in *Proc. 1st Int. Cong. Sci. Stud. Ment. Defic.*, *Montpellier*, Surrey: Michael Jackson. [18]

KUSHLICK, A. and COX, C. (1970), 'Planning services for the subnormal in Wessex', in *Psychiatric Case Registers*, Dept Health and Social Security, Statistical Report Series, No. 8, London: HMSO. [18]

LACEY, C. (1966), 'Some sociological concomitants of academic streaming in a grammar school', *Brit. J. Sociol.*, 17, 3, 245–62. [37]

LAYARD, R., KING, J. and MOSER, K. (1969), *The Impact of Robbins*, London: Penguin Educational Special. [9]

LEVY, R. J. (1947), 'Institutional *v* boarding home care', *J. Personality*, 15, 233. [32]

LIGHT, R. J. and SMITH, P. V. (1969), 'Social allocation models of intelligence: a methodological inquiry', *Harvard Educational Review*, 39, 484–510. [26]

MACANDREW, C. and EDGERTON, R. (1964), 'The everyday life of institutionalised idiots', *Human Org.*, 23, 4, 312–18. [37]

MCNEMAR, Q. (1940), 'A critical examination of the University of Iowa studies of environmental influences upon the I.Q.', *Psychol. Bull.*, 37, 63–92. [26]

MARCH, J. G. (ed.), (1965), *Handbook of Organisations*, Chicago: Rand McNally & Co. [35]

MARTIN, F., BONE, M. and SPAIN, B. (1970), *Services for the Subnormal*, London: Pergamon. [37, 149]

MAXWELL, A. E. (1961), *Analysing Qualitative Data*, London: Methuen. [108, 212]

MAYNTZ, R. (1964), 'The study of organisations: a trend report and bibliography', *Current Sociology*, 13, 3, 95–156. [38]

MEADE, J. E. and PARKES, A. S. (eds) (1966), *Genetic and Environmental Factors in Human Ability*, Edinburgh: Oliver & Boyd. [26]

Ministry of Health (Scott Report) (1962), *Report on the Training of Staff of Training Centres for the Mentally Subnormal*, London: HMSO [16]

Ministry of Health (1965), *Improving the Effectiveness of the Hospital Services for the Mentally Subnormal*, London: Ministry of Health, H.M. (65)104. [16]

MONSKY, S. F. (1963), *Staffing of Local Authority Residential Homes for Children*, London: The Social Survey. [81]

MORRIS, P. (1969), *Put Away: A sociological study of institutions for the mentally retarded*, London: Routledge & Kegan Paul. [17, 20, 22, 37, 52, 55, 58, 60, 77, 149]

National Society for the Study of Education (1928), *Twenty-Seventh Year Book*, Bloomington, Ill: Public School Publishing Co. [26]

National Society for the Study of Education (1940), *Thirty-Ninth Year Book*, Bloomington, Ill: Public School Publishing Co. [26]

NIRJE, B. (1969), 'A Scandinavian visitor looks at U.S. Institutions', 51–8 in KUGEL, R.B. and WOLFENSBERGER, W. (eds), (1969). [149]

O'CONNOR, N. (1956), 'The evidence for the permanently disturbing effects of mother-child separation', *Acta. Psychol.*, 12, 174–91. [30]

PACKMAN, J. (1968), *Child Care: Needs and numbers*, London: Allen & Unwin. [12]

PARSONS, T. (1951), *The Social System*, London: Tavistock Publications. [38]

PARSONS, T., (1957), 'The mental hospital as a type of organisation', in GREENBLATT, M., LEVINSON, D. J. and WILLIAMS, R. H. (eds) (1957). [38]

PARSONS, T. (1960), *Structure and Process in Modern Societies*, London: Cass. [35, 179]

PASTORE, N. (1949), *The Nature-Nurture Controversy*, New York: King's Crown Press, Columbia Univ. [26]

PERROW, C. (1965), 'Hospitals: Technology, structure and goals', in MARCH J. G. (ed.), (1965). [37, 38]

PINNEAU, S. R. (1955), 'The infantile disorders of hospitalism and anaclitic depression', *Psychol. Bull.*, 52, 429–62. [33]

POLSKY, H. W. (1962), *Cottage Six: The social system of delinquent boys in residential treatment*, New York: Russell Sage Foundation. [37]

POLSKY, H. W., and CLASTER, D. S. (1968), *The Dynamics of Residential Treatment*, Chapel Hill: Univ. of N. Carolina Press. [37]

PUGH, D. S., HICKSON, D. J., HININGS, C. R., MACDONALD, K. M., TURNER, C. and LUPTON, T. (1963), 'A conceptual scheme for organisational analysis' *Admin. Sci. Q.*, 8, 3, 289–315. [47]

# REFERENCES

RAPOPORT, R. N. (1960), *Community as Doctor*, London: Tavistock Publications. [39]

RAYNES, N. V. (1968), 'An empirical investigation into the care of deprived children in residential organisations', unpublished Ph.D. thesis, Univ. of London. [129, 152]

RAYNES, N. V. and KING, R. D. (1968), 'The measurement of child management in residential institutions for the retarded', 637–47, in *Proc. 1st Cong. Int. Assoc. Sci. Stud. Ment. Defic.*, Montpellier, Surrey: Michael Jackson. [108]

Reports on the Work of the Children's Department, 1955–1966, London: HMSO. [16]

RHEINGOLD, H. L. (1956), 'The modification of social responsiveness in institutional babies', *Monogr. Soc. Res. Child Developm.*, 21, 1–48. [32]

RHEINGOLD, H. L. (1960), The measurement of maternal care, *Child Develop.*, 31, 565–75. [32]

ROUDINESCO, J. and APPELL, G. (1951), 'De certaines répercussions de la carence de soins maternels et de la vie en collectivité sur les enfants de 1 à 4 ans', *Bull. Soc., Med. Paris*, 67, 106. [33]

Royal Commission (1957), *Royal Commission on the Law Relating to Mental Illness and Mental Deficiency*, London: HMSO, Command 169 [20]

RUTTER, M. (1967), 'A children's behaviour questionnaire for completion by teachers: some preliminary findings', *J. Child Psychol. and Psychiat.*, 8, 1–11. [62]

RUTTER, M., TIZARD, J. and WHITMORE, K. (1970), *Education, Health and Behaviour*, London: Longman. [62]

SALISBURY, R. F. (1962), *Structures of Custodial Care: An anthropological study of a state mental hospital*, Berkeley: Univ. of Calif. Press. [38]

SCOTT, W. R. (1966), 'Some implications of organisation theory for research in health services', *Millbank Memorial Fund Q.*, 44, 4, 35–64. [38]

SCRIMSHAW, N. S. and GORDON, J. E. (eds.) (1968), *Malnutrition, Learning and Behaviour*, Cambridge, Mass.: M.I.T. Press. [39]

SIMONSEN, K. M. (1947), *Examination of Children from Children's Homes and Day Nurseries*, Copenhagen. [31]

SKEELS, H. M. (1966), 'Adult status of children with contrasting early life experiences: a follow-up study', *Child Develop. Monogr.*, 31, 3, Serial No. 105. [26, 27]

SPITZ., R. A. (1945), 'Hospitalism: an inquiry into the genesis of psychiatric conditions in early childhood', in *The Psychoanalytic Study of the Child*, New York: International Universities Press, 1, 53. [32]

SPITZ, R. A. and WOLF, K. M. (1946), 'Anaclitic depression', in *Psychoanalytic Study of the Child*, 2, 313. [31]

STANTON, A. H. and SCHWARTZ, M. S. (1954), *The Mental Hospital*, London: Tavistock Publications. [38, 40, 41]

Statistics of Education (1966), London: HMSO. [8]

SUSSER, M. (1968), *Community Psychiatry*, New York: Random House. [38]

SWIFT, D. F. and ACLUND, H. (1969), 'The sociology of education in Britain, 1960–1968: A bibliographical review', *Soc. Sci. Inform.* 8, 31–64. [37]

SYKES, G. (1958), *The Society of Captives: A study of a maximum security prison*, Princeton Univ. Press. [36]

TIZARD, J. (1962), 'Residential care of mentally handicapped children', *Proc. London Cong. Scient. Stud. of Ment. Defic.*, 2, 659–66. [37]

TIZARD, J. (1964), *Community Services for the Mentally Handicapped*, Oxford Univ. Press. [5, 22, 29, 33, 37, 95]

TIZARD, J. (1968), 'The role of social institutions in the causation prevention and alleviation of mental retardation', paper read at Peabody, N.I.M.H., Conference on Socio-Cultural Aspects of Mental Retardation, 10–12 June. [201]

TIZARD, B. and JOSEPH, A. (1970), 'Today's foundlings: A survey of young children admitted to care of Voluntary Societies in England', *New Society*, 16, 410, 585. [203]

TIZARD, B. and JOSEPH, A. (1970), 'The cognitive development of young children in residential care', *J. Child Psychol. Psychiat.*, 11, 177–86. [203]

TIZARD, J. and B. (1971), 'The social development of two-year-old children in residential nurseries' in SCHAFFER, H. R. (ed.), *The Origins of Human Social Relations*, London: Academic Press.

UDY, S. H. (1959), ' "Bureaucracy" and "rationality" in Weber's organisation theory', *Amer. Sociol. Rev.*, 24, 6, 791–5. [47]

UDY, S. H. (1965), 'The comparative analysis of organisations', in MARCH, J. G. (ed.) (1965). [41]

ULLMANN, L. P. (1967), *Institution and Outcome: A comparative study of psychiatric hospitals*, Oxford: Pergamon Press. [37, 41, 150]

VERNON, P. E. (1955), 'Presidential address: the psychology of intelligence and "G" ', *Bull. Brit. Psychol. Soc.*, 26, 1–4. [26]

VERNON, P. E. (1957), 'Intelligence and intellectual stimulation during adolescence', *Indian. Psychol. Bull.*, 2, 1–6, cited in VERNON, P. E. (1969). [28]

VERNON, P. E. (1969), *Intelligence and Cultural Environment*, London: Methuen. [28]

WEBER, M. (1957), *The Theory of Social and Economic Organisations*, London: Collier-Macmillan. [47]

WING, J. K. and BROWN, G. (1970), *Institutionalism and Schizophrenia*, Cambridge Univ. Press. [37, 41, 42, 43, 45, 200]

WOLFENSBERGER, W. (1969), 'The origin and nature of our institutional models', 59–172 in KUGEL, R. B. and WOLFENSBERGER, W. (eds) (1969). [23, 149]

WOODWORTH, R. S. (1941), *Heredity and Environment: A critical survey of recently published material on twins and foster children*, New York: Social Science Research Council. [26]

WOOTTON, B. (1959), *Social Science and Social Pathology*, London: Allen & Unwin. [33]

WOOTTON, B. (1962), 'A social scientist's approach to maternal deprivation', in AINSWORTH, M. D., *et al.* (1962). [33]

YARROW, L. J. (1961), 'Maternal deprivation: Toward an empirical and conceptual re-evaluation', *Psychol. Bull.*, 58, 459. [33]

ZETTERBERG., H. L. (ed.) (1956), *Sociology in the U.S.A.: A trend report*, Paris: UNESCO. [37]

ZUSMAN, J. (1966), 'Development of the social breakdown syndrome concept', 363–94 in GRUENBERG, E. M. (ed.) (1966). [37]

# Index

252

# The International Library of
# Sociology
## and Social Reconstruction

Edited by W. J. H. SPROTT
Founded by KARL MANNHEIM

## ROUTLEDGE & KEGAN PAUL
BROADWAY HOUSE, CARTER LANE, LONDON, E.C.4

# CONTENTS

PRINTED IN GREAT BRITAIN BY HEADLEY BROTHERS LTD
109 KINGSWAY LONDON WC2 AND ASHFORD KENT

## GENERAL SOCIOLOGY

**Brown, Robert.** Explanation in Social Science. *208 pp. 1963. (2nd Impression 1964.) 25s.*

**Gibson, Quentin.** The Logic of Social Enquiry. *240 pp. 1960. (3rd Impression 1968.) 24s.*

**Homans, George C.** Sentiments and Activities: Essays in Social Science. *336 pp. 1962. 32s.*

**Isajiw, Wsevelod W.** Causation and Functionalism in Sociology. *165 pp. 1968. 25s.*

**Johnson, Harry M.** Sociology: a Systematic Introduction. *Foreword by Robert K. Merton. 710 pp. 1961. (5th Impression 1968.) 42s.*

**Mannheim, Karl.** Essays on Sociology and Social Psychology. *Edited by Paul Keckskemeti. With Editorial Note by Adolph Lowe. 344 pp. 1953. (2nd Impression 1966.) 32s.*

— Systematic Sociology: An Introduction to the Study of Society. *Edited by J. S. Erös and Professor W. A. C. Stewart. 220 pp. 1957. (3rd Impression 1967.) 24s.*

**Martindale, Don.** The Nature and Types of Sociological Theory. *292 pp. 1961. (3rd Impression 1967.) 35s.*

**Maus, Heinz.** A Short History of Sociology. *234 pp. 1962. (2nd Impression 1965.) 28s.*

**Myrdal, Gunnar.** Value in Social Theory: A Collection of Essays on Methodology. *Edited by Paul Streeten. 332 pp. 1958. (3rd Impression 1968.) 35s.*

**Ogburn, William F.,** and **Nimkoff, Meyer F.** A Handbook of Sociology. *Preface by Karl Mannheim. 656 pp. 46 figures. 35 tables. 5th edition (revised) 1964. 45s.*

**Parsons, Talcott,** and **Smelser, Neil J.** Economy and Society: A Study in the Integration of Economic and Social Theory. *362 pp. 1956. (4th Impression 1967.) 35s.*

**Rex, John.** Key Problems of Sociological Theory. *220 pp. 1961. (4th Impression 1968.) 25s.*

**Stark, Werner.** The Fundamental Forms of Social Thought. *280 pp. 1962. 32s.*

## FOREIGN CLASSICS OF SOCIOLOGY

**Durkheim, Emile.** Suicide. A Study in Sociology. *Edited and with an Introduction by George Simpson. 404 pp. 1952. (4th Impression 1968.) 35s.*

— Professional Ethics and Civic Morals. *Translated by Cornelia Brookfield. 288 pp. 1957. 30s.*

**Gerth, H. H.,** and **Mills, C. Wright.** From Max Weber: Essays in Sociology. *502 pp. 1948. (6th Impression 1967.) 35s.*

**Tönnies, Ferdinand.** Community and Association. *(Gemeinschaft und Gesellschaft.) Translated and Supplemented by Charles P. Loomis. Foreword by Pitirim A. Sorokin. 334 pp. 1955. 28s.*

3

## SOCIAL STRUCTURE

**Andreski, Stanislav.** Military Organization and Society. *Foreword by Professor A. R. Radcliffe-Brown. 226 pp. 1 folder. 1954. Revised Edition 1968. 35s.*

**Cole, G. D. H.** Studies in Class Structure. *220 pp. 1955. (3rd Impression 1964.) 21s. Paper 10s. 6d.*

**Coontz, Sydney H.** Population Theories and the Economic Interpretation. *202 pp. 1957. (3rd Impression 1968.) 28s.*

**Coser, Lewis.** The Functions of Social Conflict. *204 pp. 1956. (3rd Impression 1968.) 25s.*

**Dickie-Clark, H. F.** Marginal Situation: A Sociological Study of a Coloured Group. *240 pp. 11 tables. 1966. 40s.*

**Glass, D. V.** (Ed.). Social Mobility in Britain. *Contributions by J. Berent, T. Bottomore, R. C. Chambers, J. Floud, D. V. Glass, J. R. Hall, H. T. Himmelweit, R. K. Kelsall, F. M. Martin, C. A. Moser, R. Mukherjee, and W. Ziegel. 420 pp. 1954. (4th Impression 1967.) 45s.*

**Jones, Garth N.** Planned Organizational Change: An Exploratory Study Using an Empirical Approach. *About 268 pp. 1969. 40s.*

**Kelsall, R. K.** Higher Civil Servants in Britain: From 1870 to the Present Day. *268 pp. 31 tables. 1955. (2nd Impression 1966.) 25s.*

**König, René.** The Community. *232 pp. Illustrated. 1968. 35s.*

**Lawton, Denis.** Social Class, Language and Education. *192 pp. 1968. (2nd Impression 1968.) 25s.*

**McLeish, John.** The Theory of Social Change: Four Views Considered. *About 128 pp. 1969. 21s.*

**Marsh, David C.** The Changing Social Structure in England and Wales, 1871-1961. *1958. 272 pp. 2nd edition (revised) 1966. (2nd Impression 1967.) 35s.*

**Mouzelis, Nicos.** Organization and Bureaucracy. An Analysis of Modern Theories. *240 pp. 1967. (2nd Impression 1968.) 28s.*

**Ossowski, Stanislaw.** Class Structure in the Social Consciousness. *210 pp. 1963. (2nd Impression 1967.) 25s.*

## SOCIOLOGY AND POLITICS

**Barbu, Zevedei.** Democracy and Dictatorship: Their Psychology and Patterns of Life. *300 pp. 1956. 28s.*

**Crick, Bernard.** The American Science of Politics: Its Origins and Conditions. *284 pp. 1959. 32s.*

**Hertz, Frederick.** Nationality in History and Politics: A Psychology and Sociology of National Sentiment and Nationalism. *432 pp. 1944. (5th Impression 1966.) 42s.*

**Kornhauser, William.** The Politics of Mass Society. *272 pp. 20 tables. 1960. (3rd Impression 1968.) 28s.*

**Laidler, Harry W.** History of Socialism. Social-Economic Movements: An Historical and Comparative Survey of Socialism, Communism, Co-operation, Utopianism; and other Systems of Reform and Reconstruction. *New edition. 992 pp. 1968. 90s.*

**Lasswell, Harold D.** Analysis of Political Behaviour. An Empirical Approach. *324 pp. 1947. (4th Impression 1966.) 35s.*

**Mannheim, Karl.** Freedom, Power and Democratic Planning. *Edited by Hans Gerth and Ernest K. Bramstedt. 424 pp. 1951. (3rd Impression 1968.) 42s.*

**Mansur, Fatma.** Process of Independence. *Foreword by A. H. Hanson. 208 pp. 1962. 25s.*

**Martin, David A.** Pacificism: an Historical and Sociological Study. *262 pp. 1965. 30s.*

**Myrdal, Gunnar.** The Political Element in the Development of Economic Theory. *Translated from the German by Paul Streeten. 282 pp. 1953. (4th Impression 1965.) 25s.*

**Polanyi, Michael.** F.R.S. The Logic of Liberty: Reflections and Rejoinders. *228 pp. 1951. 18s.*

**Verney, Douglas V.** The Analysis of Political Systems. *264 pp. 1959. (3rd Impression 1966.) 28s.*

**Wootton, Graham.** The Politics of Influence: British Ex-Servicemen, Cabinet Decisions and Cultural Changes, 1917 to 1957. *316 pp. 1963. 30s.*
Workers, Unions and the State. *188 pp. 1966. (2nd Impression 1967.) 25s.*

## FOREIGN AFFAIRS: THEIR SOCIAL, POLITICAL AND ECONOMIC FOUNDATIONS

**Baer, Gabriel.** Population and Society in the Arab East. *Translated by Hanna Szöke. 288 pp. 10 maps. 1964. 40s.*

**Bonné, Alfred.** State and Economics in the Middle East: A Society in Transition. *482 pp. 2nd (revised) edition 1955. (2nd Impression 1960.) 40s.*
Studies in Economic Development: with special reference to Conditions in the Under-developed Areas of Western Asia and India. *322 pp. 84 tables. 2nd edition 1960. 32s.*

**Mayer, J. P.** Political Thought in France from the Revolution to the Fifth Republic. *164 pp. 3rd edition (revised) 1961. 16s.*

## CRIMINOLOGY

**Ancel, Marc.** Social Defence: A Modern Approach to Criminal Problems. *Foreword by Leon Radzinowicz. 240 pp. 1965. 32s.*

**Cloward, Richard A., and Ohlin, Lloyd E.** Delinquency and Opportunity: A Theory of Delinquent Gangs. *248 pp. 1961. 25s.*

**Downes, David M.** The Delinquent Solution. A Study in Subcultural Theory. *296 pp. 1966. 42s.*

**Dunlop, A. B.,** and **McCabe, S.** Young Men in Detention Centres. *192 pp. 1965. 28s.*

**Friedländer, Kate.** The Psycho-Analytical Approach to Juvenile Delinquency: Theory, Case Studies, Treatment. *320 pp. 1947. (6th Impression 1967). 40s.*

**Glueck, Sheldon** and **Eleanor.** Family Environment and Delinquency. *With the statistical assistance of Rose W. Kneznek. 340 pp. 1962. (2nd Impression 1966.) 40s.*

**Mannheim, Hermann.** Comparative Criminology: a Text Book. *Two volumes. 442 pp. and 380 pp. 1965. (2nd Impression with corrections 1966.) 42s. a volume.*

**Morris, Terence.** The Criminal Area: A Study in Social Ecology. *Foreword by Hermann Mannheim. 232 pp. 25 tables. 4 maps. 1957. (2nd Impression 1966.) 28s.*

**Morris, Terence** and **Pauline,** assisted by **Barbara Barer.** Pentonville: A Sociological Study of an English Prison. *416 pp. 16 plates. 1963. 50s.*

**Spencer, John C.** Crime and the Services. *Foreword by Hermann Mannheim. 336 pp. 1954. 28s.*

**Trasler, Gordon.** The Explanation of Criminality. *144 pp. 1962. (2nd Impression 1967.) 20s.*

## SOCIAL PSYCHOLOGY

**Barbu, Zevedei.** Problems of Historical Psychology. *248 pp. 1960. 25s.*

**Blackburn, Julian.** Psychology and the Social Pattern. *184 pp. 1945. (7th Impression 1964.) 16s.*

**Fleming, C. M.** Adolescence: Its Social Psychology: With an Introduction to recent findings from the fields of Anthropology, Physiology, Medicine, Psychometrics and Sociometry. *288 pp. 2nd edition (revised) 1963. (3rd Impression 1967.) 25s. Paper 12s. 6d.*
The Social Psychology of Education: An Introduction and Guide to Its Study. *136 pp. 2nd edition (revised) 1959. (4th Impression 1967.) 14s. Paper 7s. 6d.*

**Homans, George C.** The Human Group. *Foreword by Bernard DeVoto. Introduction by Robert K. Merton. 526 pp. 1951. (7th Impression 1968.) 35s.*
Social Behaviour: its Elementary Forms. *416 pp. 1961. (3rd Impression 1968.) 35s.*

**Klein, Josephine.** The Study of Groups. *226 pp. 31 figures. 5 tables. 1956. (5th Impression 1967.) 21s. Paper 9s. 6d.*

**Linton, Ralph.** The Cultural Background of Personality. *132 pp. 1947. (7th Impression 1968.) 18s.*

**Mayo, Elton.** The Social Problems of an Industrial Civilization. With an appendix on the Political Problem. *180 pp. 1949. (5th Impression 1966.) 25s.*

**Ottaway, A. K. C.** Learning Through Group Experience. *176 pp. 1966. (2nd Impression 1968.) 25s.*

**Ridder, J. C. de.** The Personality of the Urban African in South Africa. A Thematic Apperception Test Study. *196 pp. 12 plates. 1961. 25s.*

**Rose, Arnold M.** (Ed.). Human Behaviour and Social Processes: an Inter-actionist Approach. *Contributions by Arnold M. Rose, Ralph H. Turner, Anselm Strauss, Everett C. Hughes, E. Franklin Frazier, Howard S. Becker, et al. 696 pp. 1962. (2nd Impression 1968.) 70s.*

**Smelser, Neil J.** Theory of Collective Behaviour. *448 pp. 1962. (2nd Impression 1967.) 45s.*

**Stephenson, Geoffrey M.** The Development of Conscience. *128 pp. 1966. 25s.*

**Young, Kimball.** Handbook of Social Psychology. *658 pp. 16 figures. 10 tables. 2nd edition (revised) 1957. (3rd Impression 1963.) 40s.*

## SOCIOLOGY OF THE FAMILY

**Banks, J. A.** Prosperity and Parenthood: A study of Family Planning among The Victorian Middle Classes. *262 pp. 1954. (3rd Impression 1968.) 28s.*

**Bell, Colin R.** Middle Class Families: Social and Geographical Mobility. *224 pp. 1969. 35s.*

**Burton, Lindy.** Vulnerable Children. *272 pp. 1968. 35s.*

**Gavron, Hannah.** The Captive Wife: Conflicts of Housebound Mothers. *190 pp. 1966. (2nd Impression 1966.) 25s.*

**Klein, Josephine.** Samples from English Cultures. *1965. (2nd Impression 1967.)*
1. Three Preliminary Studies and Aspects of Adult Life in England. *447 pp. 50s.*
2. Child-Rearing Practices and Index. *247 pp. 35s.*

**Klein, Viola.** Britain's Married Women Workers. *180 pp. 1965. (2nd Impression 1968.) 28s.*

**McWhinnie, Alexina M.** Adopted Children. How They Grow Up. *304 pp. 1967. (2nd Impression 1968.) 42s.*

**Myrdal, Alva and Klein, Viola.** Women's Two Roles: Home and Work. *238 pp. 27 tables. 1956. Revised Edition 1967. 30s. Paper 15s.*

**Parsons, Talcott and Bales, Robert F.** Family: Socialization and Interaction Process. *In collaboration with James Olds, Morris Zelditch and Philip E. Slater. 456 pp. 50 figures and tables. 1956. (3rd Impression 1968.) 45s.*

**Schücking, L. L.** The Puritan Family. *Translated from the German by Brian Battershaw. 212 pp. 1969. About 42s.*

7

## THE SOCIAL SERVICES

**Forder, R. A.** (Ed.). Penelope Hall's Social Services of Modern England. *288 pp. 1969. 35s.*

**George, Victor.** Social Security: Beveridge and After. *258 pp. 1968. 35s.*

**Goetschius, George W.** Working with Community Groups. *256 pp. 1969. 35s.*

**Goetschius, George W. and Tash, Joan.** Working with Unattached Youth. *416 pp. 1967. (2nd Impression 1968.) 40s.*

**Hall, M. P., and Howes, I. V.** The Church in Social Work. A Study of Moral Welfare Work undertaken by the Church of England. *320 pp. 1965. 35s.*

**Heywood, Jean S.** Children in Care: the Development of the Service for the Deprived Child. *264 pp. 2nd edition (revised) 1965. (2nd Impression 1966.) 32s.*

An Introduction to Teaching Casework Skills. *190 pp. 1964. 28s.*

**Jones, Kathleen.** Lunacy, Law and Conscience, 1744-1845: the Social History of the Care of the Insane. *268 pp. 1955. 25s.*

Mental Health and Social Policy, 1845-1959. *264 pp. 1960. (2nd Impression 1967.) 32s.*

**Jones, Kathleen and Sidebotham, Roy.** Mental Hospitals at Work. *220 pp. 1962. 30s.*

**Kastell, Jean.** Casework in Child Care. *Foreword by M. Brooke Willis. 320 pp. 1962. 35s.*

**Morris, Pauline.** Put Away: A Sociological Study of Institutions for the Mentally Retarded. *Approx. 288 pp. 1969. About 50s.*

**Nokes, P. L.** The Professional Task in Welfare Practice. *152 pp. 1967. 28s.*

**Rooff, Madeline.** Voluntary Societies and Social Policy. *350 pp. 15 tables. 1957. 35s.*

**Timms, Noel.** Psychiatric Social Work in Great Britain (1939-1962). *280 pp. 1964. 32s.*

Social Casework: Principles and Practice. *256 pp. 1964. (2nd Impression 1966.) 25s. Paper 15s.*

**Trasler, Gordon.** In Place of Parents: A Study in Foster Care. *272 pp. 1960. (2nd Impression 1966.) 30s.*

**Young, A. F., and Ashton, E. T.** British Social Work in the Nineteenth Century. *288 pp. 1956. (2nd Impression 1963.) 28s.*

**Young, A. F.** Social Services in British Industry. *272 pp. 1968. 40s.*


## SOCIOLOGY OF EDUCATION

**Banks, Olive.** Parity and Prestige in English Secondary Education: a Study in Educational Sociology. *272 pp. 1955. (2nd Impression 1963.) 32s.*

**Bentwich, Joseph.** Education in Israel. *224 pp. 8 pp. plates. 1965. 24s.*

**Blyth, W. A. L.** English Primary Education. A Sociological Description. *1965. Revised edition 1967.*

1. Schools. *232 pp. 30s. Paper 12s. 6d.*
2. Background. *168 pp. 25s. Paper 10s. 6d.*

**Collier, K. G.** The Social Purposes of Education: Personal and Social Values in Education. *268 pp. 1959. (3rd Impression 1965.) 21s.*

**Dale, R. R.,** and **Griffith, S.** Down Stream: Failure in the Grammar School. *108 pp. 1965. 20s.*

**Dore, R. P.** Education in Tokugawa Japan. *356 pp. 9 pp. plates. 1965. 35s.*

**Edmonds, E. L.** The School Inspector. *Foreword by Sir William Alexander. 214 pp. 1962. 28s.*

**Evans, K. M.** Sociometry and Education. *158 pp. 1962. (2nd Impression 1966.) 18s.*

**Foster, P. J.** Education and Social Change in Ghana. *336 pp. 3 maps. 1965. (2nd Impression 1967.) 36s.*

**Fraser, W. R.** Education and Society in Modern France. *150 pp. 1963. (2nd Impression 1968.) 25s.*

**Hans, Nicholas.** New Trends in Education in the Eighteenth Century. *278 pp. 19 tables. 1951. (2nd Impression 1966.) 30s.*
  Comparative Education: A Study of Educational Factors and Traditions. *360 pp. 3rd (revised) edition 1958. (4th Impression 1967.) 25s. Paper 12s. 6d.*

**Hargreaves, David.** Social Relations in a Secondary School. *240 pp. 1967. (2nd Impression 1968.) 32s.*

**Holmes, Brian.** Problems in Education. A Comparative Approach. *336 pp. 1965. (2nd Impression 1967.) 32s.*

**Mannheim, Karl** and **Stewart, W. A. C.** An Introduction to the Sociology of Education. *206 pp. 1962. (2nd Impression 1965.) 21s.*

**Morris, Raymond N.** The Sixth Form and College Entrance. *231 pp. 1969. 40s.*

**Musgrove, F.** Youth and the Social Order. *176 pp. 1964. (2nd Impression 1968.) 25s. Paper 12s.*

**Ortega y Gasset, José.** Mission of the University. *Translated with an Introduction by Howard Lee Nostrand. 86 pp. 1946. (3rd Impression 1963.) 15s.*

**Ottaway, A. K. C.** Education and Society: An Introduction to the Sociology of Education. *With an Introduction by W. O. Lester Smith. 212 pp. Second edition (revised). 1962. (5th Impression 1968.) 18s. Paper 10s. 6d.*

**Peers, Robert.** Adult Education: A Comparative Study. *398 pp. 2nd edition 1959. (2nd Impression 1966.) 42s.*

**Pritchard, D. G.** Education and the Handicapped: 1760 to 1960. *258 pp. 1963. (2nd Impression 1966.) 35s.*

**Richardson, Helen.** Adolescent Girls in Approved Schools. *Approx. 360 pp. 1969. About 42s.*

**Simon, Brian** and **Joan** (Eds.). Educational Psychology in the U.S.S.R. *Introduction by Brian and Joan Simon. Translation by Joan Simon. Papers by D. N. Bogoiavlenski and N. A. Menchinskaia, D. B. Elkonin, E. A. Fleshner, Z. I. Kalmykova, G. S. Kostiuk, V. A. Krutetski, A. N. Leontiev, A. R. Luria, E. A. Milerian, R. G. Natadze, B. M. Teplov, L. S. Vygotski, L. V. Zankov. 296 pp. 1963. 40s.*

## SOCIOLOGY OF CULTURE

**Eppel, E. M., and M.** Adolescents and Morality: A Study of some Moral Values and Dilemmas of Working Adolescents in the Context of a changing Climate of Opinion. *Foreword by W. J. H. Sprott. 268 pp. 39 tables. 1966. 30s.*

**Fromm, Erich.** The Fear of Freedom. *286 pp. 1942. (8th Impression 1960.) 25s. Paper 10s.*

The Sane Society. *400 pp. 1956. (4th Impression 1968.) 28s. Paper 14s.*

**Mannheim, Karl.** Diagnosis of Our Time: Wartime Essays of a Sociologist. *208 pp. 1943. (8th Impression 1966.) 21s.*

Essays on the Sociology of Culture. *Edited by Ernst Mannheim in co-operation with Paul Kecskemeti. Editorial Note by Adolph Lowe. 280 pp. 1956. (3rd Impression 1967.) 28s.*

**Weber, Alfred.** Farewell to European History: or The Conquest of Nihilism. *Translated from the German by R. F. C. Hull. 224 pp. 1947. 18s.*

## SOCIOLOGY OF RELIGION

**Argyle, Michael.** Religious Behaviour. *224 pp. 8 figures. 41 tables. 1958. (4th Impression 1968.) 25s.*

**Nelson, G. K.** Spiritualism and Society. *313 pp. 1969. 42s.*

**Stark, Werner.** The Sociology of Religion. A Study of Christendom.
Volume I. Established Religion. *248 pp. 1966. 35s.*
Volume II. Sectarian Religion. *368 pp. 1967. 40s.*
Volume III. The Universal Church. *464 pp. 1967. 45s.*

**Watt, W. Montgomery.** Islam and the Integration of Society. *320 pp. 1961. (3rd Impression 1966.) 35s.*

## SOCIOLOGY OF ART AND LITERATURE

**Beljame, Alexandre.** Men of Letters and the English Public in the Eighteenth Century: 1660-1744, Dryden, Addison. Pope. *Edited with an Introduction and Notes by Bonamy Dobrée. Translated by E. O. Lorimer. 532 pp. 1948. 32s.*

**Misch, Georg.** A History of Autobiography in Antiquity. *Translated by E. W. Dickes. 2 Volumes. Vol. 1, 364 pp., Vol. 2, 372 pp. 1950. 45s. the set.*

**Schücking, L. L.** The Sociology of Literary Taste. *112 pp. 2nd (revised) edition 1966. 18s.*

**Silbermann, Alphons.** The Sociology of Music. *Translated from the German by Corbet Stewart. 222 pp. 1963. 32s.*

## SOCIOLOGY OF KNOWLEDGE

**Mannheim, Karl.** Essays on the Sociology of Knowledge. *Edited by Paul Kecskemeti. Editorial note by Adolph Lowe. 352 pp. 1952. (4th Impression 1967.) 35s.*

**Stark, W.** America: Ideal and Reality. The United States of 1776 in Contemporary Philosophy. *136 pp. 1947. 12s.*
The Sociology of Knowledge: An Essay in Aid of a Deeper Understanding of the History of Ideas. *384 pp. 1958. (3rd Impression 1967.) 36s.*
Montesquieu: Pioneer of the Sociology of Knowledge. *244 pp. 1960. 25s.*

## URBAN SOCIOLOGY

**Anderson, Nels.** The Urban Community: A World Perspective. *532 pp. 1960. 35s.*

**Ashworth, William.** The Genesis of Modern British Town Planning: A Study in Economic and Social History of the Nineteenth and Twentieth Centuries. *288 pp. 1954. (3rd Impression 1968.) 32s.*

**Bracey, Howard.** Neighbours: On New Estates and Subdivisions in England and U.S.A. *220 pp. 1964. 28s.*

**Cullingworth, J. B.** Housing Needs and Planning Policy: A Restatement of the Problems of Housing Need and "Overspill" in England and Wales. *232 pp. 44 tables. 8 maps. 1960. (2nd Impression 1966.) 28s.*

**Dickinson, Robert E.** City and Region: A Geographical Interpretation. *608 pp. 125 figures. 1964. (5th Impression 1967.) 60s.*
The West European City: A Geographical Interpretation. *600 pp. 129 maps. 29 plates. 2nd edition 1962. (3rd Impression 1968.) 55s.*
The City Region in Western Europe. *320 pp. Maps. 1967. 30s. Paper 14s.*

**Jackson, Brian.** Working Class Community: Some General Notions raised by a Series of Studies in Northern England. *192 pp. 1968. (2nd Impression 1968.) 25s.*

**Jennings, Hilda.** Societies in the Making: a Study of Development and Redevelopment within a County Borough. *Foreword by D. A. Clark. 286 pp. 1962. (2nd Impression 1967.) 32s.*

**Kerr, Madeline.** The People of Ship Street. *240 pp. 1958. 28s.*

**Mann, P. H.** An Approach to Urban Sociology. *240 pp. 1965. (2nd Impression 1968.) 30s.*

**Morris, R. N.,** and **Mogey, J.** The Sociology of Housing. Studies at Berinsfield. *232 pp. 4 pp. plates. 1965. 42s.*

**Rosser, C.,** and **Harris, C.** The Family and Social Change. A Study of Family and Kinship in a South Wales Town. *352 pp. 8 maps. 1965. (2nd Impression 1968.) 45s.*

## RURAL SOCIOLOGY

**Chambers, R. J. H.** Settlement Schemes in Africa: A Selective Study. *Approx. 268 pp. 1969. About 50s.*

**Haswell, M. R.** The Economics of Development in Village India. *120 pp. 1967. 21s.*

**Littlejohn, James.** Westrigg: the Sociology of a Cheviot Parish. *172 pp. 5 figures. 1963. 25s.*

**Williams, W. M.** The Country Craftsman: A Study of Some Rural Crafts and the Rural Industries Organization in England. *248 pp. 9 figures. 1958. 25s. (Dartington Hall Studies in Rural Sociology.)*
The Sociology of an English Village: Gosforth. *272 pp. 12 figures. 13 tables. 1956. (3rd Impression 1964.) 25s.*

## SOCIOLOGY OF MIGRATION

**Humphreys, Alexander J.** New Dubliners: Urbanization and the Irish Family. *Foreword by George C. Homans. 304 pp. 1966. 40s.*

## SOCIOLOGY OF INDUSTRY AND DISTRIBUTION

**Anderson, Nels.** Work and Leisure. *280 pp. 1961. 28s.*

**Blau, Peter M., and Scott, W. Richard.** Formal Organizations: a Comparative approach. *Introduction and Additional Bibliography by J. H. Smith. 326 pp. 1963. (4th Impression 1969.) 35s. Paper 15s.*

**Eldridge, J. E. T.** Industrial Disputes. Essays in the Sociology of Industrial Relations. *288 pp. 1968. 40s.*

**Hollowell, Peter G.** The Lorry Driver. *272 pp. 1968. 42s.*

**Jefferys, Margot,** with the assistance of Winifred Moss. Mobility in the Labour Market: Employment Changes in Battersea and Dagenham. *Preface by Barbara Wootton. 186 pp. 51 tables. 1954. 15s.*

**Levy, A. B.** Private Corporations and Their Control. *Two Volumes. Vol. 1, 464 pp., Vol. 2, 432 pp. 1950. 80s. the set.*

**Liepmann, Kate.** Apprenticeship: An Enquiry into its Adequacy under Modern Conditions. *Foreword by H. D. Dickinson. 232 pp. 6 tables. 1960. (2nd Impression 1960.) 23s.*

**Millerson, Geoffrey.** The Qualifying Associations: a Study in Professionalization. *320 pp. 1964. 42s.*

**Smelser, Neil J.** Social Change in the Industrial Revolution: An Application of Theory to the Lancashire Cotton Industry, 1770-1840. *468 pp. 12 figures. 14 tables. 1959. (2nd Impression 1960.) 50s.*

**Williams, Gertrude.** Recruitment to Skilled Trades. *240 pp. 1957. 23s.*

**Young, A. F.** Industrial Injuries Insurance: an Examination of British Policy. *192 pp. 1964. 30s.*

## ANTHROPOLOGY

**Ammar, Hamed.** Growing up in an Egyptian Village: Silwa, Province of Aswan. *336 pp. 1954. (2nd Impression 1966.) 35s.*

**Crook, David and Isabel.** Revolution in a Chinese Village: Ten Mile Inn. *230 pp. 8 plates. 1 map. 1959. (2nd Impression 1968.) 21s.*
The First Years of Yangyi Commune. *302 pp. 12 plates. 1966. 42s.*

**Dickie-Clark, H. F.** The Marginal Situation. A Sociological Study of a Coloured Group. *236 pp. 1966. 40s.*

**Dube, S. C.** Indian Village. *Foreword by Morris Edward Opler. 276 pp. 4 plates. 1955. (5th Impression 1965.) 25s.*
India's Changing Villages: Human Factors in Community Development. *260 pp. 8 plates. 1 map. 1958. (3rd Impression 1963.) 25s.*

**Firth, Raymond.** Malay Fishermen. Their Peasant Economy. *420 pp. 17 pp. plates. 2nd edition revised and enlarged 1966. (2nd Impression 1968.) 55s.*

**Gulliver, P. H.** The Family Herds. A Study of two Pastoral Tribes in East Africa, The Jie and Turkana. *304 pp. 4 plates. 19 figures. 1955. (2nd Impression with new preface and bibliography 1966.) 35s.*
Social Control in an African Society: a Study of the Arusha, Agricultural Masai of Northern Tanganyika. *320 pp. 8 plates. 10 figures. 1963. (2nd Impression 1968.) 42s.*

**Ishwaran, K.** Shivapur. A South Indian Village. *216 pp. 1968. 35s.*
Tradition and Economy in Village India: An Interactionist Approach. *Foreword by Conrad Arensburg. 176 pp. 1966. (2nd Impression 1968.) 25s.*

**Jarvie, Ian C.** The Revolution in Anthropology. *268 pp. 1964. (2nd Impression 1967.) 40s.*

**Jarvie, Ian C. and Agassi, Joseph.** Hong Kong. A Society in Transition. *396 pp. Illustrated with plates and maps. 1968. 56s.*

**Little, Kenneth L.** Mende of Sierra Leone. *308 pp. and folder. 1951. Revised edition 1967. 63s.*

**Lowie, Professor Robert H.** Social Organization. *494 pp. 1950. (4th Impression 1966.) 50s.*

**Mayer, Adrian C.** Caste and Kinship in Central India: A Village and its Region. *328 pp. 16 plates. 15 figures. 16 tables. 1960. (2nd Impression 1965.) 35s.*
Peasants in the Pacific: A Study of Fiji Indian Rural Society. *232 pp. 16 plates. 10 figures. 14 tables. 1961. 35s.*

**Smith, Raymond T.** The Negro Family in British Guiana: Family Structure and Social Status in the Villages. *With a Foreword by Meyer Fortes. 314 pp. 8 plates. 1 figure. 4 maps. 1956. (2nd Impression 1965.) 35s.*


# DOCUMENTARY

**Meek, Dorothea L.** (Ed.). Soviet Youth: Some Achievements and Problems. *Excerpts from the Soviet Press, translated by the editor. 280 pp. 1957. 28s.*

**Schlesinger, Rudolf** (Ed.). Changing Attitudes in Soviet Russia.
2. The Nationalities Problem and Soviet Administration. Selected Readings on the Development of Soviet Nationalities Policies. *Introduced by the editor. Translated by W. W. Gottlieb. 324 pp. 1956. 30s.*

# Reports of the Institute of Community Studies

*(Demy 8vo.)*

**Cartwright, Ann.** Human Relations and Hospital Care. *272 pp. 1964. 30s.*

Patients and their Doctors. A Study of General Practice. *304 pp. 1967. 40s.*

**Jackson, Brian.** Streaming: an Education System in Miniature. *168 pp. 1964. (2nd Impression 1966.) 21s. Paper 10s.*

**Jackson, Brian** and **Marsden, Dennis.** Education and the Working Class: Some General Themes raised by a Study of 88 Working-class Children in a Northern Industrial City. *268 pp. 2 folders. 1962. (4th Impression 1968.) 32s.*

**Marris, Peter.** Widows and their Families. *Foreword by Dr. John Bowlby. 184 pp. 18 tables. Statistical Summary. 1958. 18s.*

Family and Social Change in an African City. A Study of Rehousing in Lagos. *196 pp. 1 map. 4 plates. 53 tables. 1961. (2nd Impression 1966.) 30s.*

The Experience of Higher Education. *232 pp. 27 tables. 1964. 25s.*

**Marris, Peter** and **Rein, Martin.** Dilemmas of Social Reform. Poverty and Community Action in the United States. *256 pp. 1967. 35s.*

**Mills, Enid.** Living with Mental Illness: a Study in East London. *Foreword by Morris Carstairs. 196 pp. 1962. 28s.*

**Runciman, W. G.** Relative Deprivation and Social Justice. A Study of Attitudes to Social Inequality in Twentieth Century England. *352 pp. 1966. (2nd Impression 1967.) 40s.*

**Townsend, Peter.** The Family Life of Old People: An Inquiry in East London. *Foreword by J. H. Sheldon. 300 pp. 3 figures. 63 tables. 1957. (3rd Impression 1967.) 30s.*

**Willmott, Peter.** Adolescent Boys in East London. *230 pp. 1966. 30s.*

The Evolution of a Community: a study of Dagenham after forty years. *168 pp. 2 maps. 1963. 21s.*

**Willmott, Peter** and **Young, Michael.** Family and Class in a London Suburb. *202 pp. 47 tables. 1960. (4th Impression 1968.) 25s.*

**Young, Michael.** Innovation and Research in Education. *192 pp. 1965. 25s. Paper 12s. 6d.*

**Young, Michael** and **McGeeney, Patrick.** Learning Begins at Home. A Study of a Junior School and its Parents. *About 128 pp. 1968. 21s. Paper 14s.*

**Young, Michael** and **Willmott, Peter.** Family and Kinship in East London. *Foreword by Richard M. Titmuss. 252 pp. 39 tables. 1957. (3rd Impression 1965.) 28s.*